WITHDRAWN
UTSA Libraries

Persons, Humanity,
and the Definition of Death

Persons, Humanity, and the Definition of Death

J O H N   P.   L I Z Z A

Professor
Department of Philosophy
Kutztown University of Pennsylvania
Kutztown, Pennsylvania

The Johns Hopkins University Press
Baltimore

© 2006 The Johns Hopkins University Press
All rights reserved. Published 2006
Printed in the United States of America on acid-free paper

2 4 6 8 9 7 5 3 1

The Johns Hopkins University Press
2715 North Charles Street
Baltimore, Maryland 21218-4363
www.press.jhu.edu

Library of Congress Cataloging-in-Publication Data

Lizza, John P., 1957–
Persons, humanity, and the definition of death / John P. Lizza.
p. ; cm.
Includes bibliographical references and index.
ISBN 0-8018-8250-8 (hardcover : alk. paper)
1. Death—Proof and certification. 2. Brain death. 3. Humanity. 4. Persons.
5. Medical jurisprudence.
[DNLM: 1. Death. 2. Brain Death. 3. Jurisprudence.
4. Personhood. 5. Public Policy. W 820 L789p 2006] I. Title.
RA1063.L59 2006
614′.1—dc22
2005013360

A catalog record for this book is available from the British Library.

For Kristiina, Kiira, Sofia, and Elena

Contents

Preface

This work challenges the "biological paradigm" of death that has provided the theoretical grounding for acceptance of "brain death" as death. Whereas the paradigm treats human or personal death as a strictly biological matter, I hope to show that human or personal death is no less a metaphysical, ethical, and cultural matter than a biological one and that such considerations are necessary to justify any particular definition and criteria for death.

In chapter 1, I examine how the biological paradigm of death came to be established. Some of the initial work on whether to expand the criteria for determining death to include neurological criteria did not endorse the paradigm. Instead, there was recognition that defining death and choosing criteria for its determination were not strictly biological matters. Certain beliefs in the paradigm of death were needed, however, to justify acceptance of the "whole-brain" neurological criterion for determining death as opposed to retaining only the traditional circulatory and respiratory criteria or moving to a higher-brain or consciousness-related criterion for death.

Three different biological definitions of death have been proposed by theorists who work within the paradigm: Bernat, Culver, and Gert (1981); Becker (1975); and Rosenberg (1983). In chapter 2, I show how these proposals fail because they need to be supplemented by a more ontologically and ethically informed view of the nature of what dies (i.e., the human being or person).

In chapter 3, I discuss how alternative concepts of personhood affect the definition of death. Simplifying the account somewhat, I distinguish three concepts of personhood: (1) a species concept that strictly identifies the person with the human organism or body;[1] (2) a qualitative or functionalist concept that identifies the person with certain abilities and qualities of awareness;[2] and (3) a substantive concept that treats the person not as some qualitative or functional specification of some more basic kind of thing (e.g., a human organism) but as a primitive substance that has psychological and corporeal characteristics.[3] Relying on these distinctions, I show how parties in the debate over the definition of death have used different concepts of person and thus have been talking past each other by proposing definitions of death for different kinds of things. In particular, critics of the consciousness-related, neurological formulation of death have relied on concepts of person that would be rejected by proponents of that formulation: persons as qualitative specifications of human organisms or persons as identical to human organisms. Since advocates of the consciousness-related formulation of death are not committed to either of these views of personhood, these critics commit the fallacy of attacking a straw man. I clarify the substantive concept of person that may be invoked in the consciousness-related formulation of death and argue that, in this view and contra Bernat, Culver, and Gert, persons have always been the kind of thing that can literally die. I conclude by suggesting that the discussion of defining death needs to focus on which approach to personhood makes the most sense metaphysically and morally.

In the second section of chapter 3, I show how the conceptual basis for accepting a consciousness-related, neurological criterion for death has been obscured by some of the main proponents of that criterion—for example, Robert Veatch (1975, 1988) and Green and Wikler (1980). These theorists have accepted a problematic, qualitative or functionalist view of persons, instead of the more defensible, substantive view that provides the correct conceptual grounding for a consciousness-related definition and criterion of death. Although the loss of consciousness, rather than the loss of organic integration, has long been considered a possible justification for accepting brain death as death, its conceptual basis has never been adequately stated. By showing how this concept of death relies on treating persons as substantive entities, I hope to put the neurological criterion for determining death on firmer conceptual grounds.

Then, in the third section of chapter 3, I consider the issue of what follows from the facts that *person* is not a univocal term and that people hold different views of personhood. I argue that these facts do not entail acceptance of a naive relativism about the definition of death. Instead, the discussion of the definition of death needs to focus on which approach to personhood makes the most sense metaphysically, morally, and culturally.

In chapters 4 to 7, I examine in more detail these three different concepts of personhood with the aim of determining which concept makes the most sense metaphysically and morally. I argue for a nonreductionist, substantive view of personhood and that acceptance of such a view, whether on dualistic or nonreductive, materialistic grounds, supports acceptance of a consciousness-related definition and criterion of death. Only the nonreductionist view of persons "takes people seriously" in an ontologically and morally charged sense. Such a view may have wide public acceptance. In chapter 8, I consider some policy consequences that would result from rejecting the biological paradigm and accepting a more pluralistic approach to defining death.

Another way of putting my critique of the medical or biological paradigm of death is to say that any strictly biological definition of death assumes some materially reductionist view about humanity or personhood. Those reductionist views conflict with what many philosophers and lay people believe about humans or persons. Thus, since any strict biological definition of death assumes some reductionist view, those who reject such views ought to reject the idea that defining death is a strictly biological matter. In short, the currently accepted biological definition of death has taken the soul out of defining death, literally for some, figuratively for others.

Trying to resolve the issue of how to treat individuals who have lost all brain function or the capacity for consciousness by appealing to biological considerations of when life ends is like trying to resolve the issue of abortion by appealing to biological considerations of when life begins. Just as that attempt has failed in the abortion debate, so does the analogous attempt fail in the debate over the definition of death. Just as we have learned that the issue of when human or personal life begins is linked to concepts of humanity and personhood that go beyond biological considerations, we should acknowledge that the issue of when human or personal life ends goes beyond biological considerations.

This book has been a long time in the making. Since completing my doctoral dissertation, *Metaphysical and Cultural Aspects of Persons*, at Columbia University in 1991, much of my research has focused on how alternative concepts of persons and personal identity affect the evaluation of issues in bioethics, particularly the problem of defining death. Some of that research has been incorporated into this work. Accordingly, I thank the editors and publishers of the book and journals in which this material initially appeared for permission to reuse it. Chapter 2 is drawn with minor changes from "Defining Death: A Biological or Cultural Matter?" in *Suffering, Death, and Identity*, edited by Robert N. Fisher, Daniel T. Primozic, Peter A. Day, and Joel A. Thompson (Amsterdam: Rodopi, 2002). Chapters 3, 6, and 7 contain material from "Defining Death for Persons and Human Organisms," *Theoretical Medicine and Bioethics* 20(5):439–53, 1999, published by Kluwer Academic Publishers and reproduced with kind permission of Springer Science and Business Media. Chapter 7 contains excerpts from "Persons and Death. What's Metaphysically Wrong with Our Current Statutory Definition of Death?" *Journal of Medicine and Philosophy* 18:351–74, 1993, reproduced by permission of Taylor & Francis, Inc., www.taylorandfrancis.com. Parts of chapters 5 and 7 are drawn from my doctoral dissertation.

I thank the Hastings Center, especially Daniel Callahan, Thomas Murray, and the librarian, Chris McKee. In 1993, as a visiting scholar at the center, I began work on the problem of defining death. Ten years later, while on sabbatical from Kutztown University of Pennsylvania, I returned to the center, where I finished the writing of this book. I cannot imagine a more pleasant and stimulating place to work. I benefited greatly from conversations with and encouragement from colleagues at the center. I also thank George Agich and the Cleveland Clinic, which I visited in 1999. Some of the research on potentiality, irreversibility, and death that I conducted there is incorporated into chapter 6.

Over the years, I have had numerous opportunities to present some of the ideas that now appear in this book and would like to express my gratitude to several institutions that provided significant support for those lectures: Kutztown University and the Pennsylvania State System of Higher Education for numerous professional development grants and sabbatical leave in 2003; the International Research and Exchange Board and the Institute for Philosophical Research of the Bulgarian Academy of Sciences for support to participate in an Advanced Workshop on Mind, Reality, and Values in Shabla, Bulgaria, in 1996; and California Polytechnic State University for the opportunity to present the paper "Medical Technology and the Meaning of Death" as part of the Philosophy at Cal Poly Lecture Series in 1995.

So many people have been gracious with their time, conversation, and correspondence on issues addressed in this work. It would be impossible to mention them all. I especially thank Jayapaul Azariah, Bernard Berofsky, Dan Brock, Assen Dimitrov, Joseph Fins, Bernard Gert, Karen Gervais, Stan van Hooft, Hide Ishiguro, Steven Lammers, Margaret Lock, Calixto Machado, Diane Michelfelder, Ted Schick, D. Alan Shewmon, Larry and Lois Steckman, Robert Taylor, Joseph Vincent, Stuart Youngner, and my colleagues and students at Kutztown University. I am indebted to Laurel Delaney for her patient proofreading of various drafts, Linda Strange for copyediting the manuscript, and Wendy Harris and the staff at the Johns Hopkins University Press for seeing the work into print. Finally, I thank my wife, Kristiina Salminen, for twenty-five years of loving support.

Persons, Humanity,
and the Definition of Death

The Biological Paradigm of Death

Advances in medical technology have posed many ethical and social problems, but perhaps none more fundamental and challenging than the problem of defining death. The development of life-sustaining technology and organ transplantation has resulted in revision, worldwide, of the legal definitions of death. In addition to the traditional criteria for determining death (i.e., irreversible cessation of circulatory and respiratory functions), most countries, including the United States, have accepted the notion that death occurs when all functions of the brain have ceased.

These revisions have generated continuing debate over whether the law should define death in terms of loss of "higher" and "lower" brain functions.[1] This question becomes especially difficult when we consider the moral and legal status of anencephalics[2] and individuals in a permanent vegetative state (PermVS),[3] assuming that they have no potential for higher-brain functions but retain lower, autonomic brainstem functions. Why should we not consider as "dead" individuals who lack the potential for consciousness, thought, feeling, and every other mental function? There is also renewed debate about whether the move to a whole-brain criterion should have been made in the first place. Cases of postmortem pregnancy in which whole-brain-dead pregnant women have been sustained for several hours to several months (Field et al. 1988; Bernstein et al. 1989; Anstötz 1993) and the extraordinary case in which a male with no brain function has been sustained for more than fourteen years (Shewmon 1998b) raise issues about whether death has really occurred.

These cases, then, raise fundamental issues about the concepts of life and death that are central to our norms and values. Critical methodological questions also arise. Is death a strictly biological concept and, therefore, within the province of biologists to define? Or does defining death involve metaphysical and moral claims? Is the definition of death more a matter of metaphysical, moral, or social decision than a biological fact to be discovered?

The "received" view on these methodological issues is perhaps most concisely stated in seven assumptions that make up what James Bernat (2002, 329–32) calls the "paradigm of death":

1. *Death* is a nontechnical word that we all use correctly to refer to the cessation of an organism's life.
2. *Death* is a biological concept and not one that is socially constructed; the event of death is an objective, immutable biological fact that can be studied, described, and modeled but cannot be altered or contrived.
3. *Death* should be univocal across higher animal species and not defined idiosyncratically for *Homo sapiens*.
4. Because the concept of death is biological, it may be applied directly only to organisms: all living organisms must die and only living organisms can die. Any other use of *death*, such as the death of a person or culture, is a metaphorical use of the term.
5. "Alive" and "dead" are the only two fundamental underlying states of any organism. All organisms must be alive or dead; none can be both or neither.
6. Death is an event and not a process.
7. Death is irreversible.

According to Bernat, this paradigm frames the parameters of any sensible discussion about the definition and criteria of death: "Failure to first agree on the paradigm of death leads to category incongruence and thus to intractable disagreement. For example, failure to accept that death is fundamentally a biological phenomenon precludes concurrence on any unitary definition or criterion of death" (Bernat 2002, 329).

In addition to (1) to (7), I suggest that two other assumptions have been part of the paradigm:

8. Acceptance of neurological criteria for determining death does not introduce a new concept of death but is simply a new way of determining when death, as traditionally understood, occurs.
9. There is a sharp distinction between asking when a person is dead and when a person should be allowed to die. Defining death is an objective biological matter and does not involve ethical decisions about whether or when to terminate treatment for living human beings or about which lives are worth preserving.

Assumption (8) is consistent with the idea that death is an unalterable biological phenomenon. No matter what medical advances or cultural constructions may take place, death remains the same biological fact. Death cannot be altered, even though it may be possible to discover new criteria for determining when it occurs. There are not and cannot be any new ways of dying. Assumption (9) also supports the idea that defining death is fundamentally a biological matter and not one that is informed by ethical or social considerations. Just as any other biological issue is decided by scientific, not ethical, investigation, so too is the definition of death.

In his seminal discussion of scientific paradigms, Thomas Kuhn (1970) notes that the central beliefs that make up such paradigms are mutually supporting. Indeed, there is a kind of circularity of mutual support within the paradigm itself. This is evident in the nine assumptions listed above. In addition to the connections mentioned among (8), (9), and other beliefs in the paradigm, (1), (3), (4), and (5) are dependent on (2). Assumption (4) depends explicitly on the truth of (2). Because (1) asserts that the ordinary use of *death* refers to the cessation of an "organism's" life and this ordinary use of *death* is not "metaphorical," it also presupposes (2). Assumption (3) also presupposes (2) because, if death were a socially constructed concept and not strictly biological, there might be reason for thinking that the meaning of death for *Homo sapiens* could differ from that for other species. Because (5) asserts that death is one of two possible states "of any organism," it also assumes that death is a biological concept that is literally appropriate only to organisms. Assumption (5) also presupposes (6): if death were a process rather than an event, then there might not be a clear distinction in some cases whether an organism was alive or dead.

In addition, (1) and (4) may be given as a reason for (2). If the ordinary, nontechnical and nonmetaphorical use of *death* correctly refers to the cessation of the life of *organisms*, then death may indeed be a biological event and not one that can be socially altered or contrived. Insofar as (3) emphasizes what is biologically common to all higher animal species and not what may be distinctive about human beings, it supports the idea that death is a biological concept. Finally, if death is one of two fundamental, underlying states of any organism, as stated in (5), then death may be fundamentally a biological phenomenon.

I agree with Bernat that this set of assumptions has framed the debate over the definition and criteria of death and has led to acceptance of the whole-brain neurological criterion for death. It was accepted by the highly influential 1981 President's Commission for the Study of Ethical Problems in Medicine and Biomedical and Behavioral Research. It has been defended by many theorists who have worked on the issue of brain death (Bernat, Culver, and Gert 1981; Lamb 1985; Russell 2000; Korein 1997; Becker 1975; Rosenberg 1983; Feldman 1992; Taylor 1997). It has provided the conceptual basis throughout most of the world for accepting "brain death" as death. This book, however, aims to challenge the paradigm, more specifically the set of interrelated and mutually supporting assumptions (1) to (5), (8), and (9). I have less to say about (6) and (7), although I will comment on both in the course of this work.

The paradigm can be summarized as the belief that death is fundamentally or strictly a biological phenomenon. The definition and criteria of death are thus understood to be within the province of biologists or physicians. The alternative to this medical or biological paradigm of death is to think that death is a metaphysical, ethical, and cultural phenomenon *in as equally a fundamental sense* as it is a biological phenomenon. The definition and criteria of death are therefore as much matters involving metaphysical reflection, moral choice, and cultural acceptance as they are biological facts to be discovered. For these reasons, we should not look for a unitary definition or criterion of death. This is an implication that I believe enriches us, not one that should be obfuscated and avoided by pretending that the definition and criteria of death are strictly biological or medical matters. It promotes an understanding of our nature as beings that are open-ended rather than timelessly fixed, as having an active role in creating and determining the bounds of our being rather than being passive recipients of physical forces. Moreover, it's true.

Although I hope to offer fresh arguments for this thesis, the thesis itself is not new. Hans Jonas got it right very early in the debate over the definition of death, when he wrote that "the decision to be made [on how to treat individuals who have lost all brain function] . . . is an axiological one and not already made by clinical fact" (Jonas 1974, 136). Although Jonas thought we should admit a certain "vagueness" in defining human life and death, he believed that any answer to whether individuals who have lost all brain function should be treated as "dead" must be ultimately settled by "a definition of man and what life is human" (136).

As Karen Gervais also observes, "Since the human being is ontologically complex, in the sense that the human can be regarded as one among other living organisms, or as distinctive among organisms (i.e., as a person), a definition of death rests on one or the other of these ways of regarding the human being" (Gervais 1989, 14). She argues that "the choice of a perspective on the human being is value laden, an ethical choice that must be given an ethical evaluation" and that "a full justification of a concept of death requires that we cite the characteristics of the individual that we now think it appropriate to treat as dead, and justify the claim that those characteristics should be determinative that a human being has died" (14–15). She concludes that the task of fully justifying any concept of human death requires ontological and moral argumentation.

More recently, D. Alan Shewmon concurs: "The scope of physiologically cogent debate surrounding 'brain death' has narrowed to a single nonphysiological issue: the concept of 'personhood.' Unfortunately, this controversy is a purely metaphysical and definitional one which cannot be resolved with further empirical data. Western society seems to be rapidly approaching the stage where the moment of death will be determined not so much by objective bodily changes as by the philosophy of personhood of those in charge. If this trend continues, philosophers, not doctors, will ultimately (though indirectly) be the ones determining the timing of death for purposes of death certificates" (Shewmon 1997, 84–85).[4]

Bernat (1999) asserts that, because life is fundamentally a biological phenomenon, defining death is fundamentally biological. The problem with this claim is that it is incomplete. We are not interested in when life as such ceases but in when the life of certain kinds of beings ceases. The theoretical underpinning of my claim is the Aristotelian idea, reiterated and developed most notably in the work of the contemporary philosopher David Wiggins (1980, 15), that "everything that exists is a *this such.*" In this "Thesis of the Sortal Dependency of Individuation" (paraphrasing Wiggins), any judgment that a thing that is alive is the same thing that dies has no chance of being true unless two conditions are satisfied: (1) there exists some known or unknown answer to the question "same *what?*" and (2) this answer affords some principle by which the entities of this particular kind—some kind containing things that are such as to live and die—may be traced through space and time and reidentified as one and the same. The corollary to this principle is that everything that ceases to exist ceases to exist as a *this such.* Thus, if death is a form of ceasing to exist, we can maintain that the death of the human being or person is fundamentally or strictly biological only if we accept that the human being or person, what dies or ceases to exist, is fundamentally or strictly identical to a biological being.[5] If there are moral, metaphysical, and cultural aspects of human beings or persons that are essential to their nature, then the death of these entities, their ceasing to exist, cannot be understood in purely biological terms.[6] In the history of philosophy and religion, there are many reasons for rejecting the strict identification of the human being or person with a biological organism. Dualism and nonreductive materialism are two examples. In these and other views, the death of the human being or person is no less a metaphysical and moral phenomenon than a biological one.

In sum, the attempt to reduce the matter of defining death to a clinical or biological decision is a fundamental mistake when coming to terms with individuals who have lost all brain function or have irreversibly lost the capacity for consciousness. This view sterilizes the debate about the definition of death of its ontological and ethical complexities. Worse, those who reject the point of Jonas, Gervais,

Shewmon, and others commit the all too common error in bioethics of assuming that what is fundamentally a metaphysical and ethical issue can be resolved by medicine or biology.

I believe that the problem of defining death has persisted because the more fundamental ontological and ethical issues have never been adequately addressed, and a "conceptual dissonance" has resulted from an inability to reconcile a strictly biological definition of human or personal death with views about humanity and personhood that are not strictly biological. This dissonance has been particularly evident in the Japanese debate over brain death. Although some have understood the necessity of providing ontological and moral rationale, there has been insufficient attention to these issues in the bioethical literature and certainly in the public realm. In this work, I hope to cast greater light on the ontological and ethical issues that underlie the debate over the definition of death and to bring these issues more to the fore for further critical reflection and debate.

CHAPTER ONE

Establishment of the Biological Paradigm

Before presenting my arguments for challenging the biological paradigm, I shall examine whether and to what extent the assumptions in the paradigm were made in the early work on defining death, when neurological criteria for death were first introduced. While it might be claimed that these assumptions were accepted long before the modern discussion of the definition and criteria of death, there is no evidence for such a claim. Indeed, I believe human death has always been understood as a metaphysical, ethical, and cultural phenomenon as fundamentally as it was understood as a biological phenomenon. The emphasis on the biological aspects of death over its metaphysical, ethical, and cultural aspects in arriving at a definition of death is a modern invention.

How did the "paradigm" come to be established? The modern challenge to articulate a definition and criteria of death was instigated by advances in medical technology and organ transplantation in the early 1950s and 1960s.[1] In the 1950s, the increased use of ventilators created clinical situations in which the patient's heart would beat spontaneously, but the patient had no discernible brain activity and respiration was mechanically sustained. To some, it seemed that these patients were more dead than alive. If so, the traditional criterion of determining death on the basis of cessation of circulation and respiration was inadequate.

These cases also raised the issue of whether the death of the person had to necessarily coincide with the death of the human organism. As in Locke's hypothetical case of the prince and cobbler switching bodies (Locke [1694] 1975, bk. II, ch. 27, para. 15), in which the life history of the person could diverge from the life history of the human organism, some people regarded these clinical situations as actual cases in which the life histories of the person and human organism diverged. These cases also raised the issue of what it is that literally dies. Do persons, understood as in some sense distinct from human organisms, "die"? Or is death something that can only be literally predicated to human organisms or to persons understood as identical to human organisms, as assumed in the biological paradigm?

In the 1960s, advances in organ transplantation techniques and some unusual legal cases provided additional impetus to rethinking the legal definition of death. Since organ transplantation requires well-preserved organs and is facilitated by removing organs from the donor as soon as possible, there was interest in declaring death at the earliest possible moment. Adopting a neurological or brain-based criterion for determining death would enable death to be declared earlier in some clinical situations.

The unusual legal cases included one in New York in which a woman was assaulted, became comatose, and required ventilator support. When a physician later removed her from the ventilator, the person accused of the assault argued that the doctor's action, not the assault, caused the woman's death. The physician argued that the woman was already dead when he shut down the ventilator (Beauchamp and Perlin 1978, 3). A second case, in Virginia, involved a laborer who fell and suffered a massive head injury on May 24, 1968. After undergoing surgery, the patient, Bruce Tucker, was placed on a ventilator. He had a flat electroencephalograph "with occasional artifact." An organ transplantation team later removed Tucker's heart. The surgeons argued that Tucker had died, even though Virginia law at the time defined death as "a total stoppage of the circulation of the blood, and a cessation of the animal and vital functions consequent thereto such as respiration and pulsation." In a suit brought by Tucker's family challenging the surgeons' action, the Virginia court found that the surgeons were not guilty of wrongful death of the decedent. This was interpreted by some as the court's endorsement of a neurological criterion for determining death (Veatch 1972, 1978).

In 1967/68, under the leadership of Henry Beecher, the Ad Hoc Committee of the Harvard Medical School to Examine the Definition of Brain Death (1968) proposed "irreversible coma" (a permanently nonfunctioning brain) as a new criterion of death. This committee was extremely influential in promoting adoption of a neurological criterion for death and establishment of the medical paradigm for the definition of death. As Martin Pernick (1999, 13–14) points out, Beecher thought that the matter of defining death should be left in medical hands and that philosophers, in particular, had little to contribute.

In 1970, Kansas became the first state to legally adopt the recommendation of the Harvard Committee. Many other states, however, did not adopt the new criterion, and thus arose the problem that someone could be dead in Kansas but alive, for example, in the neighboring state of Missouri.

To address this problem, the 1981 President's Commission for the Study of Ethical Problems in Medicine and Biomedical and Behavioral Research was charged with proposing a uniform statutory definition of death that could be adopted by all states in the union. The result of the commission's efforts was the Uniform Determination of Death Act, which holds, "An individual who has sustained either (1) irreversible cessation of circulatory and respiratory functions, or (2) irreversible cessation of all functions of the entire brain, including the brainstem, is dead" (President's Commission 1981, 2). By 1994 every state and the District of Columbia had either judicially or legislatively adopted the provisions of the act.[2] New Jersey is exceptional in having subsequently enacted a "conscience clause," which specifies that, for individuals who do not accept any neurological criterion for determining death, only the traditional criterion of cessation of circulation and respiration need apply.[3] Some Orthodox Jews and American Indians, for example, reject the neurological criterion on religious grounds. New York allows some discretion but is less explicit about exceptions to the declaration of death on the basis of neurological criteria. It allows but does not require physicians to accommodate family views on the definition of death (Veatch 1999, 138). Such legal provisions provide some early acknowledgment that the definition of death goes beyond biological or medical considerations.

Some of the early work on the problem of defining and determining death explicitly recognized that the definition or concept of death was *not* a strictly biological matter. For example, in "Refinements in Criteria for the Determination of Death: An Appraisal," a 1972 report by the Task Force on Death and Dying of the Institute of Society, Ethics, and the Life Sciences (the institute now known as the Hastings Center), the definition or concept of death was recognized as a philosophical question that the task force was unable to resolve. Instead, the task force offered what it hoped would be refinements in the criteria for determining death that would be acceptable to people with various concepts of death.

Similarly, as Karen Gervais (1986, 8–10) points out, when the Ad Hoc Committee of the Harvard Medical School formally introduced a neurological criterion for determining death in 1968, the committee proposed "irreversible coma" as a new criterion for death and suggested clinical tests for its determination. The committee's report says little, if anything, about the *definition* of death for which the criterion was proposed. Also, as Martin Pernick (1999, 12) observes, Beecher shifted back and forth between endorsing the loss of consciousness and endorsing the loss of bodily integration as the conceptual foundation for the whole-brain diagnostic criterion that the committee eventually proposed. Indeed, the committee's characterization of the criterion as "irreversible coma" reflected this ambiguity, as the term had been used in the past to describe the condition of individuals in deep coma or persistent vegetative state (Joynt 1984).

The assumption that death is fundamentally or strictly a biological phenomenon was also not explicit in an early article by Alexander Capron and Leon Kass (1972) and in the influential 1981 report of the President's Commission. In their early work, Capron and Kass state that the basic concept of death is "fundamentally a philosophical matter," not a biological one. They then give three examples of what they called "philosophical" definitions or concepts of death: " 'permanent cessation of the integrated functioning of the organism as a whole,' 'departure of the animating or vital principle,'. . . [and] 'irreversible loss of personhood'" (Capron and Kass 1972, 102).

While Capron and Kass identify these definitions as "philosophical," the first is a strictly biological one. The other two are "philosophical" in that they invoke concepts such as "vital principle" and "personhood" that may not be understood solely in biological terms. However, Capron and Kass go on to say that such "abstract definitions offer little concrete help in determining whether a person has died, but they may very well influence how one goes about devising standards and criteria" (102).

In almost identical language, the report of the President's Commission states that "the *basic concept* of death is fundamentally a philosophical matter" (55).[4] The commission then went on to give the same examples of "philosophical" conceptions of death. However, the commission cautioned that "broader formulations would lead down arcane philosophical paths which are at best somewhat removed from practical application in the formulation of law" (President's Commission 1981, 56).

Let me say at the outset that I am troubled by the inconsistency in this view: that even though defining death is "fundamentally a philosophical matter," we should not journey down the "arcane" philosophical paths. While such a concern might be appropriate to some degree, given the practical urgency of the commission's charge, it provides no rationale for why the rest of us should stick our heads in the sand and fail to address the philosophical issues.

Although the commission acknowledged that defining death goes beyond biological considerations, the assumption that death is fundamentally a biological matter was later endorsed by the commission's acceptance of the strictly biological concept or definition of death, the "permanent cessation of the functioning of the organism as a whole." Its discussion of the "whole-brain" formulation of death noted: "On this view, death is that moment at which the body's physiological system ceases to constitute an integrated whole. Even if life continues in individual cells or organs, life of the organism as a whole requires complex integration and without the latter, a person cannot properly be regarded as alive" (33).

In addition, the President's Commission claimed that its acceptance of the "whole-brain" neurological criterion of death did not introduce a new concept of death but merely provided another means for determining when death, as traditionally understood, occurs (41).[5] The rationale offered by the commission was that it viewed death, in the traditional sense, to mean the loss of integration of the organism as a whole. Just as the irreversible loss of heart and lung functions marks the loss of integration of the organism as a whole, so, too, the commission argued, the loss of all brain functions marks the loss of organic integration. Death occurs when functions essential to the maintenance of the organism as an organism, as opposed to a collection of organic parts, permanently cease. Thus, the brain is understood as the essential control center for the integration of the organism as a whole.

Acceptance of this strictly biological definition of death and other assumptions in the paradigm was necessary because the President's Commission needed to respond to two problematic classes of individuals that challenged the criteria. The first class, which at the time of the commission's report was more hypothetical than real, consists of artificially sustained human beings with no brain functions, such as artificially sustained pregnant women who have lost all brain functions but are maintained on "life support" to allow the fetus to gestate long enough so that it can be removed by cesarean delivery (Field et al. 1988; Bernstein et al. 1989; Anstötz 1993). This class would also include the extraordinary case reported by D. Alan Shewmon (1998b) in which a male with no brain functions has been sustained for more than fourteen years. Critics of the neurological criterion for death argue that such individuals are still alive, as they retain organic integration and have not lost syntropy (Jonas 1974; Becker 1975; Truog 1997; Halevy and Brody 1993; Brody 1999; Grant 2000; Seifert 1993; Byrne et al. [1982/83] 2000; Taylor 1997; Veatch 1982, 1992; Gervais 1986; Shewmon 1997, 1998a, 1998b, 2004b; Wikler 1995). To rule out this class of counterexamples to the proposed criteria, the President's Commission relied on the strictly biological concept of death as the loss of the integration of the organism as a whole. The commission argued that such individuals are collections of organic parts rather than integrated organisms. James Bernat (2002) makes essentially the same argument.

The second problematic class consists of anencephalics and individuals in a permanent vegetative state (PermVS). Proponents of a consciousness-related definition of death argue that persons or human beings who have sustained an irreversible loss of consciousness and every other mental function are dead (Engelhardt 1975; Veatch 1975, 1988, 1993; Green and Wikler 1980; Gervais 1986; Zaner 1988; Lizza 1991, 1993b; Machado 1995; McMahan 1995). A breathing human body is not itself a person or human being. Lacking the potential or capacity for consciousness and every other mental function, anencephalics and individuals in PermVS are merely breathing bodies. The person that the anencephalic might have been never lived, and the person who has irreversibly lost consciousness and every other mental function has died.[6] To rule out these individuals as counterexamples to the whole-brain criterion, the commission relied on the idea that anencephalics and individuals in PermVS are still integrated organisms because their brainstem functions coordinate circulation and respiration to maintain the organism as a whole. In doing this, the commission rejected the concept of death as the irreversible loss of personhood or personal identity.

It should be no surprise that, despite its avowal to offer only criteria for determining death and avoid the philosophical issues that come with formulating a definition or concept of death, the commission would be forced at some point to endorse a particular concept of death. When problematic cases force us to question the criteria, we need to reflect back on and define more carefully what the criteria are for—that is, what we are trying to determine by use of the criteria.[7] By analogy, suppose a college admissions committee is looking for good prospective students. It may devise selection criteria with some idea of what a good prospective student is, but the committee may receive applications that challenge the criteria. The committee is then forced to reexamine its understanding of a good prospective student and define its concept more clearly.

Challenges to the whole-brain criterion of death have thus come from two sides: (1) those who reject any neurological criterion of death and advocate returning to reliance on only the circulatory-respiratory criterion or some other biological criterion and (2) those who support a consciousness-related criterion of death. Critics of the neurological criterion of death who are on side (1) differ among themselves in whether they accept the biological paradigm of death. For example, Lawrence Becker (1975) and Robert Taylor (1997) reject the neurological criterion of death but accept the belief that defining death is a strictly biological matter. In their view, individuals who have lost all brain function may still retain organic integration, albeit through artificial support, and are therefore still alive. Shewmon (1997, 1998a, 1998b, 1999, 2001, 2004b) and Josef Seifert (1993), however, reject the assumption that defining death is a strictly biological matter, as well as the neurological criteria for death. Like Becker and Taylor, Shewmon and Seifert believe that individuals who have lost all brain function may still retain their organic integration, but they view the continuation of organic integration as evidence that an immaterial soul is still present in the body. Thus, Shewmon and Seifert accept the traditional, theological definition of death as the separation of the soul from the body. Arguing from a Catholic perspective that understands the human being as a union of body and spirit, they reject biologically reductionist definitions of human life and death.

Because Becker, Taylor, Shewmon, and Seifert reject neurological criteria for death, they hold that artificially sustained whole-brain-dead human organisms, anencephalics, and individuals in PermVS are living human beings—but their justification for doing so differs. What is significant for Becker and Taylor is that these individuals retain their organic integration. Even if these individuals have no potential for consciousness or any other mental function, they continue to assimilate oxygen, metabolize food, eliminate wastes, and maintain a relative homeostasis. Entropy has not set in. For Shewmon and Seifert, however, this organic integration is significant not in itself but because it is indicative of the continued presence of the soul. Shewmon, for example, holds that these individuals retain the potential for consciousness, intellect, and will, since such potential is not dependent on a functioning brain: "the potency for these specifically human functions resides—ultimately—in the organism and not the organ" (Shewmon 1997, 74).

Critics of the whole-brain criterion who are on side (2) reject the biological paradigm of death. For example, Engelhardt (1975), Green and Wikler (1980), Gervais (1986), McMahan (1995, 2002), and Lizza (1991, 1993b, 1999a, 1999b) distinguish the life of the person from that of the human organism and argue that organic integration is insufficient for the continued life of persons. The artificially sustained whole-brain dead, anencephalics, and individuals in PermVS may be living human beings or living beings of some other kind (e.g., "humanoid"), but they are not persons. In this interpretation, the person that the anencephalic might have been never existed. Persons who have irreversibly lost consciousness, such as the whole-brain dead and individuals in PermVS, are considered to have died. Because the death of a person may occur before the organism has lost its organic integration, or before entropy has set in, personal death cannot be defined in such strictly biological terms.

In addition to adopting the strictly biological definition of death as the loss of integration of the organism as a whole, proponents of the whole-brain criterion of death, such as Bernat, Culver, and Gert (1981), Bernat (2002), Capron and Lynn (1982), Downie (1990), Lamb (1985), and Russell (2000), have invoked other beliefs within the paradigm to respond to the challenges from those who advocate a consciousness-related criterion and those who reject any neurological criterion. For example, one reason for rejecting the irreversible loss of consciousness in the definition and criterion of death is that it seems to introduce a special, or "idiosyncratic," meaning of death for persons or human beings that differs from that for other organisms. Although proponents of a strictly biological definition of death agree that there cannot be a special definition or concept of death for persons or human organisms, they differ on whether there is a univocal definition of death for *all* organisms. For example, Bernat (2002) accepts that the definition or concept of death for higher-order organisms may differ from that for lower-order organisms. In contrast, Fred Feldman (1992) claims that "death" is a biological concept univocal for all living organisms.

I will have more to say in the following chapter about whether acceptance of any neurological criterion for death introduces a new concept of death for human beings or persons, as Veatch (1993), Gervais (1986), Lock (2002), and others have claimed, or whether it is simply a new means of determining when death, as traditionally understood, occurs. I will side with Veatch, Gervais, and Lock on this question. At this point, I simply wish to show how the claim that the meaning of death cannot vary according to the kind of thing that dies has been used to support and has thus become a part of the biological paradigm of death. Also, although proponents of the whole-brain neurological criterion for death claim that any concept of death that is not strictly biological departs from our ordinary usage and understanding of the term, they differ over what they take to be the common understanding. Bernat apparently believes that, in our ordinary concept and understanding of death, *death* may mean something different for higher-order organisms than for lower-order organisms, whereas Feldman rejects this claim. My view is that the meaning of death may vary with the kind of thing that dies and that we have always understood and treated the death of persons and human organisms differently from that of other organisms.[8] This special treatment derives from our special nature—that is, (1) the importance of the potential for consciousness in our understanding of human life and what it means to be human, (2) the moral status accorded to persons or human beings, and (3) our nature as social and cultural beings.

In this chapter, I have tried to show how beliefs in the biological paradigm were invoked in response to challenges to the proposed whole-brain neurological criterion of death and to briefly map the intellectual terrain I will explore later in this work. Here, before presenting arguments (in the next chapter) for rejecting the idea that *death* is univocal for all organisms, I wish to comment on the claim by proponents of the whole-brain criterion that individuals who have lost all brain function but are receiving artificial support are not integrated organisms but merely collections of organic parts.

This claim is implausible and has been effectively critiqued by many scholars, including Becker (1975), Tomlinson (1984), Truog and Fackler (1992), Truog (1997), Halevy and Brody (1993), Seifert (1993), Byrne et al. ([1982/83] 2000), Taylor (1997), Veatch (1982, 1992), Gervais (1986), Wikler (1995), and Shewmon (1997, 1998a, 1998b, 1999, 2001, 2004b). At bottom, individuals who have lost all brain functions but continue to function in biologically integrated ways are integrated organisms of some sort and cannot be classified as corpses. In Germany, public interest and dissatisfaction with the notion of brain death was heightened in 1992 by the Erlanger case, in which physicians tried unsuccessfully to sustain the pregnancy of a woman who had lost all brain functions. Many people questioned whether she was really dead (Schöne-Seifert 1999).

If an organism is still alive in situations such as "postmortem" pregnancy, the question arises, what is alive? It does not automatically follow that the person or human being is alive, as claimed by those who wish to maintain that death is the loss of organic integration but reject the neurological criterion for death. Advocates of a consciousness-related formulation of death do not consider such a being to be a living person. In their view, a person cannot persist through the loss of all brain functions or even the loss of just those brain functions required for consciousness and other mental functions. Thus, if an advocate of the consciousness-related formulation of death wishes to maintain that the person dies even though something is still alive, what remains alive must be a different sort of being. It must be either a human being, as distinct from a person, or a being of another sort, such as a "humanoid" or "biological artifact," by which I mean a living being that has human characteristics but falls short of being human, a form of life created by medical technology. Indeed, this may be the most sensible thing to say about such a living being. Whereas a person is normally transformed into a corpse at his or her death, technology has intervened in this natural process and has made it possible for the person to die in new ways. Instead of a person's death resulting in remains in the form of an inanimate corpse, a person's remains can now take the form of a living being devoid of the capacity for consciousness and any other mental function.

Hans Jonas rejected neurological criteria for death, but he referred to the body of the whole-brain dead and the irreversibly comatose as a "residual continuance of the subject." He also thought that this being was "still entitled to some of the sacrosanctity accorded to such a subject by the laws of God and men" and that "that sacrosanctity decrees that it must not be used as a mere means" (Jonas 1974, 139). What Jonas means by "residual continuance of the subject" is unclear. His phrase is vague, perhaps reflecting his view that there is vagueness about defining death and we should give vagueness its due. Nevertheless, to refer to these bodies as a "residual continuance of the subject" suggests that something short of the subject persists. For could not the same be said about a corpse? We treat human corpses with respect and do not use them simply as a mere means. Even when bodies are used for organ transplantation, they are not treated as mere means. We respect the wishes of the deceased subject and the family and cannot simply use the body in whatever way we want. Indeed, the respect accorded to persons carries over in various ways, even after death.

My point is that the new cases brought about by medical technology pose new challenges. We grope for language to describe what exists. We try to integrate our metaphysical and ethical beliefs into an appropriate response. Ultimately, what we call such living beings and how we treat them will depend on broader ontological and ethical considerations and on how consistent what we say about these beings is with what we say about persons, human beings, corpses, rights, respect, and so forth. The challenge to probe the philosophical and ethical issues concerning the nature and meaning of death cannot be avoided.

CHAPTER TWO

Defining Death

Beyond Biology

Proponents of a consciousness-related or "higher-brain" formulation of death hold that the capacity for consciousness is essential to the life of a human being or person and that death occurs when a human being or person loses this capacity (Engelhardt 1975; Veatch 1975, 1988; Green and Wikler 1980; Gervais 1986; Lizza 1993b; McMahan 1995, 2002). Advocates of this view understand consciousness and other cognitive functions as dependent on or identical to certain higher-brain functions, and when those brain functions cease, the human being or person dies. Individuals in a permanent vegetative state (PermVS), who have irreversibly lost all higher-brain functions but have retained functions of the brainstem such as the regulation of breathing and heartbeat, are therefore considered dead. A breathing human body is not itself a living human being or person, and without higher-brain functions, individuals in PermVS are merely breathing bodies.

The "received" whole-brain formulation of death, accepted by the President's Commission for the Study of Ethical Problems in Medicine and Biomedical and Behavioral Research (1981), Bernat, Culver, and Gert (1981, 1982a), and many others, understands brain function as significant because it is necessary for the integration of the human organism. The brain is the controlling center of the organism, responsible for the autonomous regulation of circulatory and respiratory functions. Without a functioning brain, the human being or person loses its organic integration and thus dies. Although the loss of all brain functions, including those of the brainstem, entails the loss of consciousness, the loss of consciousness itself is not what makes the loss of all brain functions significant for the death of the human being or person.

Thus, individuals in PermVS are not dead, since their functioning brainstem enables them to retain their organic integration.

Critics of the consciousness-related formulation of death have pointed out that acceptance of a consciousness-related neurological criterion would introduce not only a new criterion for determining death but a radically new concept of death — a special meaning of death for human beings or persons that differs from that for other species (President's Commission 1981; Bernat, Culver, and Gert 1982a; Culver and Gert 1982, 182–84; Lamb 1985; Feldman 1992; Russell 2000). These critics claim that *death* should mean the same thing whether applied to human beings or to other species. If there is a univocal definition of death for all organisms, it cannot have anything to do with an organism's loss of consciousness, as many living things that die are never conscious. For example, Fred Feldman claims that *death* is a biological concept univocal for all living organisms. According to Feldman, there is no reason to think that the word *died* has one meaning in the sentence "J.F.K. died in November 1963" and a different meaning in the sentences "The last dodo bird died in April 1681" or "My oldest Baldwin apple tree died during the winter of 1986" (Feldman 1992, 19). Feldman thus denies that there is any special meaning of death for persons or higher-order organisms. Moreover, he thinks this univocal trans-species meaning of death is part of our ordinary understanding of death; thus, acceptance of a special consciousness-related formulation of death would depart from our ordinary usage and understanding of the term. This same argument has been used by David Lamb (1985), Tom Russell (2000), Bernat, Culver, and Gert (1982a, 1982b), Capron and Lynn (1982), Downie (1990), and the President's Commission (1981) in support of a strictly biological definition of death.

In this chapter, I challenge the notion of a univocal, strictly biological definition of death for all organisms. I critically examine three such definitions and show how each entails either treating some individuals as dead who are clearly alive or treating some individuals as alive who are clearly dead.

I first look at the rationale behind the President's Commission's acceptance of the whole-brain criterion of death and at the actual biological definition of death accepted by the commission and later explicitly formulated by Bernat, Culver, and Gert: "the permanent cessation of the functioning of the organism as a whole." I argue that consideration of the locked-in syndrome and other hypothetical cases shows this definition to be inadequate. Bernat and Gert have acknowledged the difficulties with the definition they initially proposed. These difficulties, however, have led them to revise the definition in a way that implies that the loss of brain function is significant for the death of a human being or person not because those functions are connected to the loss of organic integration but because they are connected to consciousness. Thus, there is a special meaning of death for human be-ings, persons, and perhaps other higher-order species that is tied to the irreversible loss of consciousness and other mental functions.

I then consider two alternative, biological definitions of death, proposed by Lawrence Becker (1975) and by Jay Rosenberg (1983). A consideration of PermVS and the hypothetical case of an artificially sustained, decapitated human body shows that their biological definitions also fail. Any definition of death for human beings or persons is thus tied to conceptions of humanity and personhood that go beyond biological taxonomy and biological definitions of life and death. Building on what I find sensible in Rosenberg's account, I propose a definition of death that is explic-itly linked to conceptions of humanity and personhood.

DEATH AS THE LOSS OF ORGANIC INTEGRATION

Although the President's Commission endorsed a neurological criterion of death in addition to the traditional circulatory and respiratory criteria, the commission maintained that the neurological criterion did not introduce a new concept of death but merely provided another means for determining when death, as traditionally un-derstood, occurs (President's Commission 1981, 41). The commission's rationale was that it viewed death in the traditional sense as meaning the loss of integration of the organism as a whole. Just as the permanent loss of heart and lung functions marks the loss of integration of the organism as a whole, so the loss of all brain function marks the loss of organic integration. Death occurs when functions essential to the maintenance of the organism as an organism, as opposed to a collection of organic parts, permanently cease. James Bernat, Charles Culver, and Bernard Gert (1982a, 1982b) later formulated this idea in terms of the following formal definition of death: "the permanent cessation of the functioning of the organism (a living biological en-tity) as a whole." These authors, later joined by Alexander Capron and Joanne Lynn (1982), argue that this definition captures what death means for any type of organism.

Stuart Youngner and Edward Bartlett (1983), however, point out that the ratio-nale behind the *definition* of death as the loss of integration of the organism as a whole does not support the whole-brain *criterion* of death that the President's Com-mission, Bernat and colleagues, and others endorse. Instead, it supports adoption of a more limited brainstem criterion, since, according to the commission, Bernat, and others, the brainstem, not neocortical structures, is responsible for integrating the organism in a life-sustaining way. In addition, because "the permanent cessation of the functioning of the organism as a whole" is supposed to capture the idea that any organism dies when it loses its internal, organic integration, it is unclear why, in this definition, higher-brain functions must cease, since those functions are not essential to the integration of the organism as a whole. Higher-brain functions would seem to be as necessary to the functioning of the organism as a whole as is, say, fingernail growth. Indeed, it is precisely because the proponents of this definition of death do not regard higher-brain functions as necessary for the integration of the organism as a whole that they do not regard individuals in PermVS as dead.

The point is that, in the trans-species definition of death accepted by the President's Commission, Bernat and colleagues, and others, higher-brain functions are unnecessary to the continued existence of the human organism as a whole, and the loss of integrative organic functions (the breakdown of the heart-lung-brainstem system) suffices for death. The problem with this definition, as Youngner and Bartlett have pointed out, is that it has the absurd implication that certain kinds of patients whom we think are alive would be "dead."

Youngner and Bartlett ask us to consider the following hypothetical case:

> After anesthetizing a 20-year-old man, an unethical physician selectively destroys all the brainstem and cerebral areas responsible for integration and regulation of the body's subsystems. In a surgical tour de force not possible in today's technology, the blood supply and the neural connections to the rest of the cerebral areas are left intact. The reticular activating system and the brainstem areas responsible for eye movement remain unaffected. Although the ability to spontaneously regulate respiration, blood pressure, temperature, hormonal balance, and other functions is lost, these functions are carefully monitored and regulated by machines and highly trained medical personnel. The patient is awake and alert, and gives meaningful responses to questions by moving and blinking his eyes.
>
> This young man has entirely lost the innate and spontaneous ability to integrate essential body subsystems. It is clear, however, that a competent medical house officer can replace those functions . . . The young man may be dying. But as long as he is conscious, no one would say that he is dead, even without the innate ability to integrate his body's subsystems. (Youngner and Bartlett 1983, 256)

Youngner and Bartlett point out that, if the loss of brain functions is a criterion for determining death because of the role those functions play in integrating the organism, we would have to say this hypothetical patient is dead.

While their case is hypothetical, it is realistic. For example, "locked-in" patients have a fairly specific and limited lesion in the ventral pons, causing de-efferentation (i.e., disconnection of the upper motor neurons in the brain from lower motor neurons in the spinal cord). The portions of the brain responsible for consciousness and cognition, however, remain intact. It is easy to imagine such a patient having additional lesions in those portions of the brain responsible for integration of vegetative functions. More specifically, suppose there are additional lesions in the medullary center, which is responsible for the initiation and maintenance of spontaneous respiration, and in the pneumotaxic center in the pons, which helps coordinate cyclic respirations. Cardiac activity is usually maintained by the dynamic balance between the nucleus of the vagus nerve located in the medulla and nuclei in the spinal cord that operate the sympathetic nervous system, but the spinal reflex circuits—without any cerebral influence—can be sufficient to maintain cardiac activity in patients who have lost all brain function (Malliani et al. 1972). Suppose, in our hypothetical patient, there is an additional lesion of the vagus nerve. Because patients who have lost all brain function have been artificially sustained for months and even longer, it is not hard to imagine sustaining a patient with locked-in syndrome who has sustained lesions in the brainstem structures involved with the regulation of cardiorespiratory function. The problem, however, is that, even though retaining consciousness, the patient has died in the trans-species sense of "the permanent cessation of the organism as a whole."[1]

If we think such patients have not died, then we need to reject the idea that the spontaneous, integrative role of the brain is what makes the loss of brain functions an adequate criterion for death. We may also have to abandon the idea of a univocal, trans-species definition of death. Recently, Bernat and Gert seem to recognize the need to embrace both consequences. For example, Bernat now states that his proposed biological definition of death applies to "higher animal species, such as vertebrates" but "may not be directly applicable to the death of the subunits of an organism, such as its cells, tissues, or organs; single-celled animals; or plants" (Bernat 2002, 330). Thus, the concept of death may vary with the kind of being that dies. "As a biological concept," however, "death should be univocal across these (higher animal) species and not defined idiosyncratically for *Homo sapiens*, because, for example, we refer to the same concept when we say that a relative has died as we do when we say that our pet dog has died" (330). Bernat then argues that acceptance of the irreversible loss of consciousness as a definition of death for persons or human beings, but not for other higher animal species, violates the requirement that death must mean the same thing for all higher animal species and offends against the common usage and understanding that death must be the same for these types of organisms.

Bernat's position is puzzling. First, he offers no general explanation of when the definition of death varies across species and when it does not. For example, why is it acceptable to have a definition of death for vertebrates that does not apply to invertebrates but unacceptable to have a definition of death for human beings or persons that does not apply to other higher animal species? How exactly does the kind of thing that dies influence the definition of death for that kind of thing? Bernat at least recognizes variation in the definition of death across species, but he never examines the details of how the kind of thing that dies affects the definition of death.

Second, even if the definition of death for a human being, a dog, and members of other higher animal species is the same, this may be because all of these organisms have some form of consciousness or sentience. Indeed, consciousness or sentience may be an essential property of these kinds of being, such that its irreversible loss would entail the death or ceasing to exist of these types of organism. This opens up several options for consciousness-related theorists. For example, they could maintain that the irreversible loss of consciousness and sentience in a dog would entail the loss of integration of the organism *as a whole* and hence would mean its death. In this view, an artificially sustained dog in PermVS may not be a dog at all. Instead, it may be the remains of a dog, a different kind of biological organism, or, perhaps more descriptively, a kind of biological artifact.

Alternatively, as I discuss in greater detail in later chapters, a consciousness-related theorist could rely on a distinction between persons and organisms such that persons are constituted by, but not identical or reducible to, living organisms. In this view, the death of the person is understood as different from the death of the organism. This distinction provides higher-brain theorists with further options, depending on what they consider to be the necessary and sufficient conditions of personhood. For example, if the capacity or potential for consciousness and sentience is necessary and sufficient for being a person but is not a necessary condition for being an organism, then the definition of the death of the person would be different from that of the organism. This particular account of personhood would classify dogs as persons, since they exhibit consciousness and sentience. In this case, the definition of death of a human being *qua* person would be the same as that of the dog *qua* person. Moreover, the definition of death of the human being *qua* organism might be the same as that of the dog *qua* organism. If more than consciousness and sentience is required for personhood, however, such as the capacity for language, rationality, or moral responsibility, then the dog would be excluded from the class of persons. The death of the human person would then be different from the death of these other kinds of being.

Gert (1995) also seems to acknowledge that the definition of death depends on the kind of thing that dies. In the light of experiments in which monkeys were kept alive for some time after their heads were severed from their bodies (R. J. White et al. 1971), Gert now believes it is necessary to include the irreversible loss of consciousness in the definition of death: "When a monkey's severed head responds to sounds and sights, claiming that it is dead alters the ordinary understanding of death far more than claiming that the monkey is still alive" (Gert 1995, 26). In order to accommodate this ordinary understanding of death, Gert amends the earlier biological definition of death that he, Bernat, and Culver proposed. Expanding on the former definition of death as "the permanent cessation of the functioning of the organism as a whole," Gert now offers the following: "An organism is dead if and only if (1) *it has permanently ceased to* function as a whole and, where applicable, (2) it has permanently lost consciousness and (3) all identifiable parts of the organism have permanently lost consciousness" (27). The amendment is needed to accommodate the fact that the decapitated monkeys were alive, even though they had ceased to function as an organic whole. Gert explains that this special meaning of death for human beings and other higher animals is necessary because "the importance of consciousness to a conscious organism has no counterpart in nonconscious animals or plants" (28).

In this amended definition of death for human beings, (1) permanent loss of integration of the organism as a whole and (2) irreversible loss of consciousness are jointly necessary and sufficient for death. Neither is individually sufficient for death. Thus, Gert continues to reject the higher-brain formulation of death: "Taking permanent loss of consciousness as sufficient for the death of a human being makes the death of a human being something *completely distinct* from the death of lower organisms" (28, emphasis added). In addition, he thinks such a definition "does not state what we ordinarily mean when we speak of death," and in support of this claim he states, "We ordinarily regard permanently comatose patients in persistent vegetative states who are sufficiently brain damaged that they have irreversibly lost consciousness as still alive" (29).

I consider in chapter 7 how Gert's argument appeals to ordinary perceptions about individuals in PermVS. For now, I wish to examine his claim that taking permanent loss of consciousness as sufficient for death would make the death of a human being "completely distinct from the death of lower organisms." There are two ways to challenge this claim. First, one might claim that, when a human being irreversibly loses consciousness, this being also loses what it means for it to be "functioning as a whole." In this view, what it means for a being to function as a whole varies with the kind of being it is. The definition of death of a human being as the irreversible loss of consciousness thus retains the idea of "ceasing to function as whole," but it includes the capacity for consciousness as essential to what it means for certain kinds of organisms to function as a whole. The problem with Gert's position is that he has tried to exclude consciousness from his account of what it means for a human being to function as a whole, while at the same time he wishes to acknowledge the importance of consciousness in the life of conscious animals. If consciousness is an *essential* human attribute, as Gert explicitly affirms, then its loss would entail the ceasing to exist (i.e., the death) of the human being. Following Aristotle (*Metaphysics* 7), an essential property is a property that something must retain as long as it continues to exist as the kind of thing it is. Thus, to exclude the capacity for consciousness as a necessary component of what it means for a human being to function as a whole is to ignore the being's essential nature.

The second way to challenge Gert's claim is to distinguish the death of the person from that of the human organism. This is the view that I favor. Persons may die even though the organisms that constituted them may continue to live. In this view, the death of the person is distinct from the death of the organism. But the death of the person cannot occur without some significant biological event taking place. Certain biological events, such as the destruction of brain functions responsible for consciousness, must occur for a person to die. Since, in part at least, the death of a person can be understood only by reference to biology, it is unclear in what sense this would make the death of the person "completely distinct" from the death of other organisms. Although, in this view, the death of the person may not coincide with the death of the organism, it is unclear that this distinction is any more problematic than the distinction that Gert accepts between the death of the organism as a whole and the death of all parts of the organism. In Gert's view, the death of the human being as a whole does not necessarily entail the death of every part of the human organism—certain organs may continue to function, fingernails may continue to grow, and so forth. The higher-brain theorist can maintain an analogous distinction: the person may die even though some of the parts that constituted the person continue to function. Indeed, the higher-brain theorist can maintain that the human organism that constituted the person may continue to function or be alive even though the person has died.

BECKER'S BIOLOGICAL DEFINITION OF DEATH

The difficulties posed by consideration of cases such as artificially sustaining a locked-in patient or even whole-brain-dead bodies have led some theorists to reject not only the idea that it is the spontaneous, integrative role of the brain that makes the loss of brain functions an adequate criterion for death. These theorists have gone on to reject neurological criteria altogether and advocate a return to reliance on only the traditional circulatory and respiratory criteria (Jonas 1974; Becker 1975; Truog 1997; Halevy and Brody 1993; Brody 1999; Grant 2000; Seifert 1993; Byrne et al. [1982/83] 2000; Quay 1993; Taylor 1997; Shewmon 1997, 1998a, 1998b; Potts, Byrne, and Nilges 2000). Thus, even though the brainstem may be destroyed, the role that it normally plays in regulating circulation and respiration can be taken over by artificial means. For these theorists, whether the brainstem functions are spontaneous is irrelevant in the determination of death. In their view, such patients are still alive.

Lawrence Becker, for example, holds that "a human organism is dead when, for whatever reason, the system of those reciprocally dependent processes which assimilate oxygen, metabolize food, eliminate wastes and keep the organism in relative homeostasis are arrested in a way which the organism . . . cannot reverse" (Becker 1975, 353). Karen Gervais rightly observes that "Becker's definition of organic death refers to the integrated function of the human body; if such functioning persists, whether spontaneously or mechanically assisted, the human being is still alive. The iron lung patient is still alive for the same reason that the totally brain-dead, respirator-driven body is alive: 'the system of . . . reciprocally dependent processes remains functional'" (Gervais 1986, 54).

Others have also invoked a kind of commonsense intuition about death that they claim underlies the traditional circulatory and respiratory criteria of death and rejects any neurological criterion. Paul Quay (1993), for example, asks us to consider two conditions of a woman whose brain has irreversibly ceased to function but who has been placed on a ventilator and other life support.

> Condition I: [The woman] . . . is profoundly unresponsive to any stimulus of pain or pleasure and is quite unable to breathe (i.e., move rib-cage or diaphragm) without the ventilator. But this patient's heart is beating. Her respiration (i.e., exchange of oxygen for gaseous wastes in the lungs and body tissues) continues. Her color is normal brown or pink. Her temperature holds its own against room-temperature, and she sweats if the room is too warm. Her kidneys continue to put out urine. Her leg will kick if the knee is tapped. More strikingly, if she is pregnant, the child continues to grow healthily in her womb. Her body, to be brief, continues to function as one single organism, though none of its functions show any influence of sensation or thought, for which the brain's activity would be needed.
>
> Condition II: After a few hours or days, a week at longest if we are speaking of an adult, even though the ventilator and the rest of the life-support system continue their activity, the heart stops; the vascular system collapses; respiration halts; the color turns bluish or gray; body-temperature approaches room-temperature; kidneys and other organs cease to function; all reflex movements disappear; the child in the womb will die if not delivered at once by Caesarian section. In a short time, rigor mortis sets in, followed by all the other usual signs of death. (Quay 1993, 1)

Quay submits that "the latter condition (II) is the condition people have always designated as 'death.' The former condition (I) has hitherto been considered the condition of a living person who is dying of some mortal injury to the brain" (1). Because conditions I and II are medically, physiologically, and biologically completely different, Quay sees no reason to label them by the same name, *death*. Only condition II can correctly be labeled *death*.

In sum, Becker's biological definition of death avoids the unacceptable implication of the idea that the irreversible loss of the brain's spontaneous, integrative functions provides an adequate criterion for determining death. In Becker's view, the locked-in patient would still be considered alive. His view also seems to meet the desideratum that human death means the same thing as the death of any other biological organism. The loss of the capacity to assimilate oxygen, maintain homeostasis, and so forth, may be what death means for any type of organism. Becker's definition also recognizes that there are significant medical, physiological, and biological differences between Quay's conditions I and II and supports the commonsense view that only individuals in condition II are dead.

Gervais (1986, 46–61) has pointed out that Becker's definition faces two major difficulties. The first is a dilemma: either Becker's proposal is logically inconsistent or it entails the unacceptable idea that death is a reversible process. Gervais argues that, when respiratory or cardiac devices are used to restore the integrative functioning of the human body, it is unclear that those functions have not been "arrested in a way which the organism . . . cannot reverse." If we say, however, that the functions *have* been arrested in a way that the organism cannot reverse, then we must say that the organism has died. But then, if we intervene mechanically to restore integrative functioning, we will have brought the dead back to life. Contrary to what Gervais holds to be the common assumption—that death is irreversible—in Becker's view, death becomes a reversible process. Gervais is unwilling to accept this idea.

The second difficulty for Becker's view, according to Gervais, "is best demonstrated with a hypothetical case. Becker's position commits us to the claim that someone who has been decapitated, yet whose body is being maintained so that those reciprocally dependent processes which assimilate oxygen, metabolize food, eliminate wastes, and keep the organism in relative homeostasis continue in stride, is alive. Surely we cannot abide this conclusion. A view such as Becker's overlooking as it does the maintenance of organic life, commits him to this absurd consequence" (Gervais 1986, 57).

Gervais's objections are strong, but not because these consequences are as absurd as she thinks. Becker could respond by asking, what is wrong with thinking that a decapitated body sustained by artificial means is a living organism? We certainly would not have a dead body in Quay's condition II. Becker could also maintain that we should give up the idea that death is irreversible. Perhaps current technology

does enable us to bring the organically dead back to life, and thus the common assumption that death is irreversible is mistaken.[2]

Even if we suppose that an artificially sustained, decapitated human body would
be alive in Becker's and Quay's biological sense, it is unclear that we would recognize
such a biological entity to be a human being or human organism. Indeed, we would
not. (If decapitation is not enough, consider also removing the limbs, so that all that
remained was a torso. If that is not enough, consider the artificial maintenance of a
system of only those human organs necessary to assimilate oxygen, metabolize food,
and eliminate wastes.) Technology would have created, in a sense, a new kind of
entity—one that fails to satisfy our concept of a human being as a natural kind.[3]

It is difficult to characterize what metaphysically would be going on if we artificially sustained a decapitated human body and held that such a living body was not
a human being but some other kind of being. Let's call this new kind of entity a
"humanoid." It has human characteristics but falls short of being human. What type
of change did the human being undergo? Did the human being die? Or should we
say that the humanoid has simply lost certain abilities and qualities that earlier made
it a human being?

At this point it is worth recalling why Bernat, Culver, and Gert reject the consciousness-related formulation of death and therewith the idea that a person in
PermVS has "died." According to them, such an assertion involves a category mistake: a failure to distinguish between (1) an organism ceasing to be a person and
(2) an organism dying:

> The alternative definition [i.e., the consciousness-related definition of death] actually
> states what it means for that person to die. *Person* is not a biological concept but rather
> a concept defined in terms of certain kinds of abilities and qualities of awareness. It is
> inherently vague. Death is a biological concept. Thus, in a literal sense, death can be
> applied directly only to biological organisms and not to persons. We do not object to
> the phrase "death of a person," but the phrase in common usage actually means the
> death of the organism which was the person . . . By our analysis, Veatch (1976) and
> others have used the phrase "death of a person" metaphorically, applying it to an or-
> ganism which has ceased to be a person but has not died. (Culver and Gert 1982, 183)

Perhaps paraphrasing the way Culver and Gert characterize the change that occurs when a human being loses personhood in PermVS, we should adopt a similar
strategy in the case of the artificially sustained, decapitated human body. Perhaps we
should distinguish between (1) an organism (the humanoid) ceasing to be a human
and (2) an organism dying. The humanoid clearly has not died in Becker's and
Quay's sense; it has just lost certain abilities and qualities necessary to be a human

being. Perhaps we should borrow further from Culver and Gert and say the following: *Human* is not a biological concept but rather a concept defined in terms of certain kinds of abilities and qualities. It is inherently vague. Death is a biological concept. Thus, in a literal sense, death can be applied directly only to biological organisms and not to humans. We do not object to the phrase "death of a human being," but the phrase in common usage actually means the death of the organism that was the human. To say that "a human being has died" is to use the phrase "death of a human being" metaphorically, applying it to an organism that has ceased to be a human being but has not died.

The point of these remarks is not to argue that we should adopt this strategy if faced with an artificially sustained, decapitated human body. Rather, it is to show that such a strategy is mistaken. Moreover, if the strategy is mistaken in this case, then it is mistaken in its analogous treatment of the change that a person undergoes when he or she sustains an irreversible loss of consciousness.

In the case of an artificially sustained, decapitated human body, we *would* say that the human being has died, and there would be nothing metaphorical about saying so. We would also insist that *human being* is a biological concept and not defined simply in terms of functions or certain abilities and qualities of life. We would also have to admit that there is some vagueness to our concept, since it would be hard to draw a sharp distinction between a human being and a humanoid.

The analogy that *humanoid* is to *human being* as *human being* is to *person* shows what is wrong with Bernat and colleagues' dismissal of the consciousness-related formulation of death. They are no more justified in their claim that proponents of the consciousness-related formulation fail to appreciate the significance of the distinction between an organism ceasing to be a person and that organism dying than we would be justified in claiming that Bernat and colleagues fail to appreciate the distinction (evident in the artificially sustained, decapitated human body) between an organism ceasing to be a human being and that organism dying. If Bernat and others are to hold that *person* is not a biological concept and that *death* applies literally only to biological organisms, then they must admit that *human being* is not a biological concept and, therefore, *death* cannot literally be applied to human beings. To avoid this difficulty, they would have to show that *human being* is not as vague a concept as *person* or that we should consider the artificially sustained, decapitated human body to be a human being and not simply a humanoid.

Both alternatives are implausible. Persons and human beings are essentially social-historical beings, and the biology of persons and human beings is not reducible to animal biology but is what Marx Wartofsky (1988, 219) has called "funny biology." Wartofsky's point is that the death of persons and human beings, unlike the death of other types of organisms, is "a socially constituted fact requiring a judgment" (219). The lines drawn between persons, humans, and humanoids, as well as the boundaries of the life and death of these biological entities, are thus determined by biological considerations as well as by metaphysical, ethical, and cultural considerations. Because these concepts are in part metaphysically, ethically, and culturally determined, they have a "vagueness" about them that is not found in pure biological taxonomy and biological definitions of life and death

Consistent with the idea that cultural judgment is involved in fixing the boundaries of our concepts of person, human, and humanoid, it seems highly implausible that our culture would support the judgment that an artificially sustained, decapitated human body was a human being. Even Orthodox Jewish law, one of the more conservative positions in the debate over the definition of death, recognizes decapitation as death (President's Commission 1981, 11).

One merit of considering the artificially sustained, decapitated human organism is that it is a hypothetical case that the general public can easily conceptualize. Intuitions about such a case may therefore reveal some assumptions about our ordinary, nontechnical understanding of death. This is especially true if there is a consensus among the public about such cases. While I have not formally surveyed people's views about such a case, I have asked many people about their intuitions. I almost universally receive the reply that they would consider themselves to have "died," even if their decapitated body were artificially maintained.

In sum, consideration of the artificially sustained, decapitated human organism, Youngner and Bartlett's hypothetical patient, and the patient in PermVS supports the idea that death cannot be defined in the strictly biological terms of the President's Commission, Bernat, Culver, and Gert, or Becker.

ANOTHER BIOLOGICAL DEFINITION OF DEATH: ROSENBERG AND TAYLOR

In Jay Rosenberg's view (1983), death is a change in kind—the living person changes into a corpse—and it can be defined as the loss of autonomous, global syntropic capacity that is permanent and irreversible. A similar biological definition of death has also been proposed by Robert Taylor (1997). I wish to retain Rosenberg's idea that death is a change in kind but suggest that there are other ways in which a person can undergo a change in kind without being changed into a corpse and that these other changes in kind constitute the death of the person. Moreover, what it means for an entity to lose its "autonomous, global syntropic capacity" is relative to the kind of entity it is.

By "syntropic capacity or ability" Rosenberg means "the capacity or ability of a living organism to preserve or even increase its structural organization through causal transactions with its environment" (Rosenberg 1983, 105). Although at times he suggests that this syntropic ability or condition of life must be "autonomous" and located in the organism "left to its own devices," he does not consider as dead those individuals whose lives are dependent on pacemakers, iron lungs, or kidney dialysis and who thus lack independent syntropic capacity. It is unclear to me what he would say about some of the cases I have presented here: PermVS, "postmortem" pregnancy, and the artificially sustained, decapitated human body. In these cases, the organism would seem to retain syntropic ability, though not independent syntropic ability, and so should not be considered "dead" in his view. These organisms do not decay and break down through interaction with the environment in the way a corpse does. The changes they undergo are not the same as the change from a living person into a corpse.

The changes that these organisms undergo are either changes in kind or changes in quality. If they are changes in quality, then, assuming with Rosenberg that death is a change in kind, death has not occurred. As noted earlier, this is the tack that Culver and Gert (1982) take in rejecting the consciousness-related brain formulation of death. For them, *person* refers to certain abilities and qualities of awareness that a human organism might have. In PermVS, the human organism has lost those abilities and qualities of awareness and has thus ceased to be a person. There has been no substantial change in kind, however, and death has not occurred. It is as if a person lost the ability to play basketball. We could say that the basketball player no longer exists but not that a death has occurred.

As I argued, a similar tack could be taken in the case in which we artificially sustain a decapitated body. We could construe a human being as a qualitative specification of some other sort of thing (e.g., humanoid) and argue that a death has not occurred in this case of decapitation. Intuitions about whether a death has occurred in this case, however, run counter to this interpretation. Most of us would say that a death has occurred. Thus, unless these intuitions are mistaken or unless we have some reason for thinking that PermVS is a qualitative change whereas decapitation is a change in kind, we should be suspicious of the claim that PermVS is merely a qualitative change in the organism and that death has not occurred.

Alternatively, the changes resulting from PermVS, loss of all brain functions, or decapitation may be changes in kind. We then need to ask whether a change in kind entails a death. Rosenberg denies this entailment. He allows for the possibility that an organism can undergo a change in number or kind without dying. He cites examples of an amoeba splitting (a change in number) and a caterpillar changing into a butterfly (a change in kind). Through these types of changes, he claims, "no life is lost." In contrast, life is not conserved through the change of kind that is death. Perhaps we should construe the changes resulting from persistent vegetative state, loss of all brain function, and decapitation as changes in which life is conserved and death does not occur. Thus, as in the above examples, a person's life might end when the person irreversibly loses higher-brain functions or all brain functions or is decapitated, but this does not necessarily mean that a death has occurred and that life has not persisted through these types of change.

There are two problems with this line of thought. First, Rosenberg's single example of a change in kind of organism without death (the metamorphosis of a caterpillar into a butterfly) is problematic, since the caterpillar is the larva of a butterfly, the earliest stage in the growth of a butterfly, and the metamorphosis is a change in the structure and habits of the insect during normal growth. No change in kind takes place. Rather, there has been a change in phase of development. Caterpillar and butterfly are phased sortals of the kind lepidoptera, rather than different substantial sortals. We are thus left with the question of whether there can be a change in kind of living organism without a death occurring.[4]

Second, it is problematic to say that life is conserved through these types of changes that a person might undergo. To say that life *simpliciter* is conserved is not helpful, since one could maintain that life is conserved even through the change of a person into a corpse. Cells in our body may continue to function even after death. Some syntropic ability at the cellular level remains.

What we need to do, therefore, is specify the kind of life that is conserved through the change. The syntropic ability of a living person or human organism is presumably not conserved through its change into a corpse. If we think the kind of life that is not conserved through death needs to be specified, however, it is far from clear that we should say the life of a person is conserved through loss of higher-brain functions and a death has not occurred with this type of change. The syntropic abilities necessary for the life of a person are different from those of other organisms, and what it means for a person to retain its systemic integrity is different from what it means for other types of living beings to retain their systemic integrity. One minimal necessary condition for the life of a person is the capacity or potential for consciousness.

The same point could be made with respect to the change that an organism undergoes when it sustains loss of all brain functions but is maintained on artificial "life" support—for example, Quay's case of maternal brain death or postmortem pregnancy. Should we construe the loss of all brain functions as a change in kind in which the life of the human organism is conserved, or should we construe it as a change in kind that is equivalent to death? The pregnant human organism retains syntropic ability, so much so that it can sustain the life of another organism—the fetus. But it seems to have lost the syntropic ability that we normally associate with a human being. It cannot sustain and increase its structural organization as normal human beings can. Thus, perhaps we should say that a death has occurred and that another kind of entity—an artifactual entity—is being sustained. Indeed, this is what we should say.

The same argument could be made in the case of an artificially sustained, decapitated human being. Rather than understanding this as a change in kind that does not entail death and in which human life is preserved, we should view it as a substantial change in kind equivalent to the death of the human being and the maintenance of some other kind of living entity.

It may be helpful to make this same point in the context of a critique of Bernat, Culver, and Gert's definition of death as the loss of integration of the organism as a whole. What we mean by *as a whole* is up for grabs. Many would argue that a person ceases to function "as a whole" when it irreversibly loses consciousness and all sentience, and therefore, contra Bernat, Culver, and Gert, the death of a person occurs when there has been an irreversible loss of consciousness and sentience, even though other biological, integrative functions remain. Thus, what it means for a person or human being to function "as a whole" is tied to views about personhood and humanity and is not something that can be settled on purely biological grounds.

The upshot of this analysis is that it requires us to specify the kind of life that lives and dies. Once we do this, we see that what constitutes the life and death of a person or a human being is tied to conceptions of personhood and humanity that go beyond biological taxonomy and biological definitions of life and death. Death can be defined as a change in kind of a living entity marked by the loss of some essential property (cf. Veatch 1978). The criteria for the death of a person or human being will therefore be determined by the loss of whatever properties are deemed essential to the nature of persons or human beings. In addition, what is deemed essential to the nature of a person or human being may vary with different metaphysical, ethical, or other cultural beliefs.

In the next three chapters, I explore how such different beliefs affect one's understanding of death. I argue that, despite variations in cultural beliefs about the nature of a person or human being, there is a remarkable consistency, at least in the Western philosophical tradition, in support of the idea that the potential for consciousness is essential for personhood. While various philosophers in the Western tradition have defined persons differently and have suggested different properties as essential to personhood, there is general agreement that the potential for consciousness is a necessary condition for being a person.

For example, Aristotle (*Nicomachean Ethics*) claimed that man is essentially a rational and social animal; Descartes ([1641] 1986), that thinking is essential to the nature of a person; Locke ([1694] 1975), that a person is an object essentially aware of its progress and persistence through time; Hume ([1739] 1978), that persons are bundles of psychological characteristics; Kant ([1781/1787] 1997; [1785] 1993), that persons are rational agents that, among other things, can synthesize experience and act on moral principles; and Sartre([1943?] 1991), that persons are self-conscious, Intentional beings. What all these philosophers have in common is the belief that some type of cognitive function is necessary for something to be a person. Any being devoid of the potential for consciousness would by implication lack each of the particular characteristics that these philosophers use to define persons.

Moreover, if the neurophysiological basis of *any* of the cognitive functions that typical persons manifest is destroyed, as in the case of individuals in PermVS (Jennet and Plum 1972; Ingvar et al. 1978; Cranford 1988; American Academy of Neurology 1989), there is an implied consensus among philosophers in the Western tradition that these entities are not persons. Finally, if death is a change in kind of living entity marked by the loss of an essential property, then the philosophical tradition strongly supports the claim that a person who has irreversibly lost consciousness has died.

Advances in medical technology make us particularly aware that human or personal death is not a strictly biological matter. Because of technological interventions in the life history of human beings and persons, human beings and persons can now die in entirely new ways. What it means to die is thus relative to the kind of thing that is alive and to the kind of medical intervention that may be applied. Technology has enabled biological entities to live in ways that previously were impossible. It is therefore reasonable to think they can die in ways that were previously impossible.

In sum, technology has created new phenomena that separate the biological and cultural aspects of death in new ways. We cannot simply look back at how the concept of death has been used in the past to determine how we should use it now. We are faced with a choice of how to project the concept in the light of new phenomena. This task involves looking not only to how we have existed in the past but to how we wish to be in the future.

CHAPTER THREE

Concepts of Person

Gilbert Meilaender claims that two competing "visions" of a person—and of the relation of person to body—have been "at war with each other since the three decades or so that bioethics has been a burgeoning movement" (Meilaender 1993, 29). The first view divorces the person from our biological nature or the history of our embodied self. It is "an ahistorical and essentialist concept of the person," which views "not the natural history of the embodied self but the presence or absence of certain capacities that makes the person" (29). Moreover, it distinguishes the class of human beings from the (narrower) class of persons and holds that "to be a person is to be, or have the capacity to be, an autonomous chooser, to take control over one's personal history" (30). Meilaender observes that this is the view that seems to be triumphing in bioethics. In the other vision of a person, the one Meilaender accepts, a person is *terra animata* or, as Paul Ramsey (1970, xiii) has put it, "an embodied soul or an ensouled body." This view draws no distinction between the class of human beings and the class of persons. As Hans Jonas (1992) maintained, we exist as living bodies, as living organisms.

Meilaender correctly observes that these different concepts of personhood have been pivotal in bioethical discussion, as different concepts of person yield different views about how certain individuals—such as human embryos and fetuses, individuals in a permanent vegetative state (PermVS), the severely demented, the "whole-brain dead," and anencephalics—should be treated. Indeed, whether a human embryo or fetus is a person has been seen by many as *the* central issue in the controversy over abortion and the status of frozen embryos. Recent attempts by antiabortion groups to introduce into law language that would refer to the fetus as a person reflect how important the concept of personhood is to the ethical and legal issues concerning the beginning of life. Significantly less attention has been paid to how disagreement about the concept of personhood affects the definition and determination of death, yet this disagreement is as critical to understanding why people differ over the definition and criteria of death as to understanding why they differ over abortion.

Meilaender oversimplifies the disagreement about concepts of personhood, however, by setting up a false dilemma. Although he correctly characterizes the first view as one that distinguishes, in some way, the class of human beings from the class of persons, there are major differences among those who accept this distinction. For example, it is one thing to hold that the potential for some cognitive function, such as consciousness, is a minimal, necessary condition of persons, and quite another thing to hold that autonomy or rationality is a necessary and sufficient condition of persons. The bounds of the classes of human beings and persons differ greatly depending on which claim we accept. Accordingly, treatment decisions will differ depending on how we classify individuals.

Thus, if some *potential* for consciousness is a necessary condition of persons, then anencephalics, individuals in PermVS, and whole-brain-dead individuals should not be considered living persons, whereas individuals with severe dementia, though they may lack rationality and autonomy, would not necessarily be ruled out of the class of living persons.[1] Prima facie, individuals with severe dementia would therefore be entitled to the kind of moral concern appropriate to any other person. In contrast, if autonomy or rationality is a necessary condition of persons, then anencephalics, individuals in PermVS, the whole-brain dead, and those with severe dementia would not be considered living persons and would not be entitled to the moral concern we normally accord to persons.

Part of the problem with Meilaender's oversimplification is that it continues to polarize the bioethical debate about treatment decisions as ultimately depending on an either/or choice about the sufficient conditions of personhood: either we believe all (and only) rational, autonomous human beings are persons or we believe any human being (organism) is a person. The reasonable, middle ground is lost in this "war." It is as if we could not adopt a more moderate position concerning one or more of the necessary conditions of persons while remaining uncertain or open-ended about the sufficient conditions.[2]

Meilaender also claims that those who distinguish the class of human beings from the (narrower) class of persons "divorce" the person from a natural, biological life history. It is unclear what Meilaender means by "divorcing" the person from a natural, biological life history. He seems to have in mind a strong sense of separation, such as that found in the common interpretation of Cartesian dualism that identifies the person with a nonphysical, mental substance (i.e., a soul) and thus separates the person from any physical body. Alternatively, he may be considering a materialistic view that identifies the person with the brain. Although retaining a connection with some physical body (i.e., the brain), this view distinguishes the person from the human body as a whole. Note that early in the debate over the definition of death, Jonas (1974) claimed that acceptance of neurological criteria for death was a reflection of acceptance of a brain/body dualism, reminiscent of the Cartesian dualism of mind and body. Jonas rejected Cartesian dualism and what he viewed as its modern version in that both identify the person with the mind rather than with the human body.

Cartesian dualism and the brain/body distinction are not the only alternative metaphysical views to identifying the person with the human organism. As we shall see, there are other views that accept that a person's life history *is* biological—that a person is *terra animata* and, if not Ramsey's "embodied soul," an embodied mind. Proponents of these views may simply disagree with Meilaender, Jonas, and others as to when the biological life history ends and may distinguish the life history of the person from that of the organism. Indeed, they may view the human body (not just the brain) to be as necessary and important as, for example, autonomy or the capacity for consciousness in determining who and what we are. In these views, a biological life history together with, for example, the potential or capacity for consciousness are held to be necessary, though perhaps not sufficient, conditions for the continued life of a person. Thus, if these theorists affirm a necessary connection between the person and the human organism, it is hard to see in what sense they are "divorcing" the person from a biological life history.

Although Meilaender is correct in his observation that the two visions of a person that he identifies have been prominent in bioethical debates, the story is more complicated. Indeed, the concepts of *person* and *personal identity* have had a long and varied history in philosophy. In recent times, especially, there has been a great deal of writing on these concepts and their application to real and hypothetical cases. This chapter thus serves as a prolegomena to the more focused discussion in subsequent chapters of different views of persons and how those views affect the definition and criteria of death.

In the first section, "Meanings of *Person*," I identify three distinct meanings or concepts of person in common discourse, philosophical theories, and the discussion of a consciousness-related definition of death. Because parties in the debate over the definition of death have employed different concepts of personhood, they have been essentially talking past each other by proposing definitions of death for different kinds of things. In particular, critics of the consciousness-related formulation of death have relied on concepts of personhood that can be rejected by proponents of that formulation, and thus the critics are attacking a straw man.

Next, in "The Consciousness-Related Formulation of Death," I show how discussion of the consciousness-related definition may have contributed to promoting the false dichotomy that Meilaender sets up. In particular, some of the main proponents of this formulation of death, such as Green and Wikler, Veatch, and Gervais, have disagreed over the concept of person. This disagreement, in turn, has led them to differ about the conceptual basis for the consciousness-related formulation of death. By explaining the disagreement and showing what is common to these theorists, I hope to put the argument for a consciousness-related formulation of death on firmer ground.

Finally, in "Persons, Philosophy, and Culture," I consider the issue of what follows from the facts that people hold different views of personhood and that *person* is not a univocal term. These facts do not entail acceptance of a naive relativism about the definition of death. Instead, a discussion of the definition of death needs to focus on which approach to personhood makes the most sense metaphysically, morally, and culturally. The remaining chapters in this work seek to contribute to that discussion.

MEANINGS OF *PERSON*

The term *person* is not univocal and has at least three distinct meanings reflected in how it is used in ordinary language as well as in the more technical language of philosophy, psychology, theology, and anthropology.[3] First, *person* is sometimes used to refer simply to the human being, body, or organism as a member of the biological species *Homo sapiens*, regardless of whether that being is alive or conscious. A sign in an elevator that reads "Maximum capacity: six persons" and references to human corpses as "dead persons" are such uses of the term.[4] Strict identification of the person with the human organism also invokes this meaning of the term. I will call this meaning of *person* its "species meaning."

In *Confrontations with the Reaper* (1992, 119), Fred Feldman invokes this meaning of *person*, which he refers to as the "biological person." Feldman argues that persons do not necessarily cease to exist after death, since they are identical to their human bodies. He admits that the way in which people continue to exist after their death is unsatisfying; nevertheless, the person "Aunt Ethel" is literally the corpse at the wake and the body that is interred. Just as dead butterflies that are carefully preserved and mounted for display are still members of their respective biological species, so the embalmed Aunt Ethel is still a member of her biological species. To be a person is to be a physical specimen of the human species. The specimen need not be alive or have any psychological characteristics.[5]

Eric Olson (1997) also endorses the view that the person is identical to the human organism, but he stipulates that the organism must be alive: a dead human organism is not a person but the remains of a person. Contrary to what Olson identifies as a common assumption in the history of Western philosophy about persons— that persons are essentially psychological beings—he argues for a nonpsychological view of persons and personal identity.[6] Persons are identical to their living bodies, regardless of whether those bodies have the potential or capacity for consciousness or any other psychological states.

Some critics of the consciousness-related, neurological formulation of death, such as Paul Ramsey and Alexander Capron, seem to accept this species meaning of person. They reject *any* distinction between persons and human organisms and identify the life history of the person with that of the human organism. In Ramsey's words (1970, 60–61), persons are "embodied souls" or "ensouled bodies." In Capron's words (1987, 8), "the accepted criterion for being considered a person" is "live birth of the product of human conception." Ramsey and Capron accept the biological definition of death as the irreversible loss of the integration of the organism as a whole, along with the whole-brain, neurological criterion for determining death. These critics thus regard individuals in PermVS and anencephalics as living persons. Death has not occurred in these cases, because the human organism (i.e., the person) has not irreversibly lost its organic integration. If all brain functions are lost, however, then the human organism (i.e., the person) has lost its organic integration and therefore has died. In this view, if we were to sustain some functions, such as heartbeat and respiration, in a whole-brain-dead human body, we would be sustaining collections of human organs rather than the person (i.e., the human organism as a whole).

Other critics of the consciousness-related, neurological formulation of death, such as Hans Jonas (1974), Josef Seifert (1993), D. Alan Shewmon (1997), and Paul Byrne and colleagues ([1982/83] 2000), also seem to accept this biological meaning of person. These critics then go on to dismiss any neurological criterion for determining death and accept only the traditional criterion of irreversible cessation of respiration and circulation. They hold that persons may irreversibly lose all brain functions but retain organic integration. In their view, such persons are still alive. For example, Shewmon (1997, 74) states, "as long as the human body is alive (from the biological perspective of somatic integrative unity) then the person is alive."

Note, however, that Shewmon accepts that any living human organism is a person only on the assumption that, by its very nature, such an organism has the potential for intellect and will. Thus, in contrast to Olson, Shewmon understands persons as essentially psychological beings, because he assumes that all living human organisms, regardless of whether they satisfy the current whole-brain criterion of death, have the potential for intellect and will. I discuss this view in more detail in chapter 6, arguing that Shewmon relies on a problematic concept of potentiality and that there is no reason to attribute the potential for intellect and will to a human being that has lost all brain function.

In the second meaning of *person*, which I call its "qualitative meaning," the term is used to designate "a character sustained or assumed in a drama or the like, or in actual life; part played; hence function, office, capacity; guise, semblance" (*Oxford English Dictionary* [Compact Ed., 1971] s.v. "person"). This qualitative meaning suggests there is something behind the "guise" or "function" that relates to the substantive reality rather than the mere appearance of the person. It also means that the reality behind the guise or role can take on many different guises or roles or present many different persons. An example of this use appears in Morton Prince's seminal work on multiple personality, when he writes, "In addition to the real, original, or normal self, the self that was born and which she [Christine Beauchamp] was intended by nature to be, she may be any one of three different persons. I say three different, because, although making use of the same body, each, nevertheless, has a distinctly different character; a difference manifested by different trains of thought, by different views, beliefs, ideals and temperament, and by different acquisitions, tastes, habits, experiences and memories" (Prince [1906] 1969, 1).

Bernat, Culver, and Gert (1981, 1982a; Culver and Gert 1982), along with other proponents of the biological paradigm of death (Downie 1990; Lamb 1985; Russell 2000), accept this qualitative meaning of person. Bernat, Culver, and Gert distinguish the person from the human organism and hold that the individual in PermVS is not a person. In their view, "*Person* is not a biological concept but rather a concept defined in terms of certain kinds of abilities and qualities of awareness. It is inherently vague. Death is a biological concept. Thus in a literal sense, it can be applied directly only to biological organisms and not to persons" (Culver and Gert 1982, 183). Thus, Culver and Gert object to characterizing individuals in PermVS as "dead" on the grounds that this would be an incorrect use of the term *dead*. They define *death* as "the permanent cessation of functioning of the organism as a whole" and claim that death is a strictly biological concept, applicable to human organisms but not to persons. Thus, they criticize the consciousness-related, neurological formulation of death as involving a metaphorical use of *death*, "applying it to an organism which has ceased to be a person but has not died" (183). In their view, *death* cannot be applied literally to persons because death is a biological concept appropriate to biological organisms, not to roles, functions, abilities, or qualities of awareness.

This "qualitative" or "functionalist" meaning of person has historical roots in John Locke's theory of personal identity and may receive support from contemporary functionalist theories of the nature of mind. Locke ([1694] 1975) distinguished the person from the human animal (organism) and questions of personal identity from those of the identity of the human animal (organism). In his discussion of the hypothetical case of a prince and cobbler swapping bodies, Locke (bk. II, ch. 27, para. 15) argued that personal identity travels with one's psychological states and memories, regardless of the substance, material or immaterial, that may underlie those psychological states and memories. Thus, if the body of the cobbler woke up one day with the psychological states and memories of the prince, and the body of the prince awoke with the psychological states and memories of the cobbler, the prince and cobbler would have swapped bodies. For Locke, personal identity over time consists of the connectedness between psychological states evident in memories.

Because the substantive matter underlying the psychological states is irrelevant to personal identity, Locke's view is a precursor to contemporary functionalist theories of the mind and personal identity. Functionalism as a philosophy of mind rejects the idea that the mind is a substantive entity, whether material (e.g., the brain) or immaterial (e.g., the soul). Instead, the mind is conceived as a function that can be described abstractly by a machine table of inputs, internal states, and outputs (Putnam [1967] 1991). While the function needs to be embodied in some medium, such as the neurophysiological processes of the brain, the function can be described independent of whatever underlies or instantiates the function. Minds are thus realizable in a variety of mediums. The medium could conceivably be nonphysical.

In the third meaning of *person*, which I call its "substantive meaning," the term is used to designate the existence, individuality, and identity of persons as substantive entities that essentially have a mind. *Person* in this sense means "the actual self or being of a man or woman; individual personality" (*Oxford English Dictionary* [Compact Ed., 1971], s.v. "person"). Personhood in this sense is what makes a particular person what she is and differentiates her from all other persons. In contrast to the "qualitative meaning," persons in this third sense are unique; they are the realities behind the guises or roles. If we substitute *person* for *self* in the above quotation from Prince and thus refer to "the real, original, or normal [person] that was born," we would be using *person* in its substantive sense. Prince was committed to the existence of persons in this sense. P. F. Strawson's definition ([1958] 1991, 1959) of a person as an individual to which we can apply both predicates that ascribe psychological characteristics (P-predicates) and predicates that ascribe corporeal characteristics (M-predicates) is another example of the use of *person* in its substantive sense. In Strawson's view, and even assuming with Bernat, Culver, and Gert that death is a biological or corporeal concept, it is neither a category mistake nor a metaphor to predicate death to persons. This substantive use of *person* is also found in the Catholic tradition, most explicitly stated in Boethius's definition of person as "an individual substance of a rational nature" (Boethius *Contra Eutychen et Nestorium* 3). Finally, commonsense usage in expressions such as "people die every day" and traditional, religious belief in personal resurrection after death are examples of a use of the concept *person* in this third sense of the term.

The substantive meaning differs from the species meaning in that it entails the person's having the capacity or potential for psychological functions. This cannot be said about a corpse or about some living members of the biological species *Homo sapiens*.[7] There are significant differences, however, among those who accept a substantive view in how they regard the nature of persons. These differences concern the nature of the substance that a person is and the psychological functions that are necessary and sufficient for persons.[8]

Substantive theories of the person may be materialistic or dualistic. Dualistic theories, such as found in Plato, in the common interpretation of Descartes, and in many religions, identify the person with an immaterial soul or mind. In this view, personal identity over time consists in the persistence of the same immaterial substance (soul). Death is understood as the separation of the soul or mind from the body (Plato *Phaedo* 64c). Ideas on when this separation occurs and what criteria are acceptable for determining death vary greatly among those who accept dualism. Thus, whereas some Christians and Jews accept the current whole-brain criterion of death, with some even accepting a consciousness-related criterion, others reject any brain-based criterion. For example, when the President's Commission for the Study of Ethical Problems in Medicine and Biomedical and Behavioral Research took testimony from Jewish religious leaders, Rabbi David Bleich rejected the whole-brain neurological criterion and "interpreted Jewish law to require a cessation of corporal blood flow, whether or not spontaneous, as a prerequisite for determining death" (President's Commission 1981, 11). In his view, as long as blood flows and respiration takes place, the body is still ensouled and death has not occurred. Rabbi Moses Tendler, in contrast, held that "the Jewish tradition would recognize complete cessation of brain function as 'physiological decapitation' and hence accept it as a basis for declaring death" (11). Indeed, as noted in chapter 1, such disagreement has resulted in New Jersey and New York enacting legal provisions to allow exceptions for individuals who reject "brain death" as death. These states, in effect, legally recognize that the matter of defining and determining death is not strictly biological.

Materialistic substantive views of the person hold that a person is a fundamental kind of substance that cannot be reduced to any other kind of thing and essentially has material and psychological properties. Materialists thus deny (1) that a person could exist separately from any material body and (2) that a person could exist simply as a material being without psychological properties. As we will see, however, materialistic substantive theories differ over the kind of material body that a person must have and whether the particular material body that a person has is necessary for the person to continue to exist.

Materialistic and immaterialistic substantive views of the person share the common belief that a person dies when a mind is no longer associated with a body or, in other words, when the psychophysical integrity of the person realized in the human body is destroyed. As noted above, death is traditionally defined as the separation of the soul or mind from the body. Dualists believe the mind or soul is not dependent on a body for its existence and thus that the mind or person is not necessarily destroyed at death. Materialists do not accept that the mind or person can exist independent of or separate from any material body. Although they agree with the dualists that death is the loss of mind from the body, they see death as the destruction of the person.

In the following chapters, I critically examine these different concepts of personhood in more detail, with the aim of showing how they can illuminate our understanding of what is at stake in the debate over the definition of death. Here, I just wish to point out that critics of the consciousness-related, neurological formulation of death have relied on concepts of personhood that may be rejected by proponents of that formulation. These critics treat persons as qualitative specifications of human organisms (e.g., Bernat, Culver, and Gert) or as identical to human organisms (e.g., Jonas, Ramsey, Capron, Seifert, and Shewmon). Advocates of a consciousness-related definition of death, however, are not committed to either of these views of personhood and may rely on a substantive view of persons, so these critics are attacking a straw man. Indeed, as I suggest in the next section, the strongest argument for a consciousness-related definition of death rests on a substantive view of personhood. In this view, and contra Bernat's "paradigm of death," persons are the kind of thing that can literally die.

THE CONSCIOUSNESS-RELATED
FORMULATION OF DEATH

The conceptual foundation for a consciousness-related formulation of death has been obscured by the way in which some of the main proponents of this formulation—Veatch, Green and Wikler, and Gervais—have presented their arguments and criticized each other's views. Disagreement among these proponents on the conceptual grounds for a consciousness-related formulation of death can be traced to their disagreement over concepts of personhood and personal identity. In my view, Karen Gervais (1986) comes closest to correctly formulating the conceptual basis for accepting a consciousness-related, neurological criterion for death: she invokes the substantive concept of the person rather than the more problematic, functionalist concept that Veatch (1992, 1993) and Green and Wikler (1980) assume or have been interpreted to assume. Also, by emphasizing how a neurological criterion of death is related to personal life and by distinguishing human biological life from human personal life, H. Tristram Engelhardt, Jr. (1978) elucidates some important aspects of the concept of death underlying acceptance of a neurological criterion.

Robert Veatch has been one of the main advocates for a consciousness-related, neurological formulation of death, but he has explicitly avoided relying on concepts of personhood or personal identity as a basis for this formulation. Like Bernat, Culver, and Gert, Veatch assumes that the only sensible concept of person is one that invokes its "qualitative meaning." Thus, in arguing in favor of a "higher-brain formulation of death," Veatch (1975, 1988, 1993) is careful to distance himself from the argument of Green and Wikler (1980), which invokes a concept of personal identity, and to present his argument as one that relies not on a view about persons but on a view about the human being.

Veatch's worry is that, in some cases of dementia, many or all theories of personhood and personal identity would hold that the person no longer exists since all trace of rationality, along with many other psychological characteristics and abilities that we associate with persons, are lost. Veatch believes that a death has not occurred in such cases.[9] In addition, he is specifically critical of Green and Wikler's argument, because their view defines death in terms of the loss of personal identity. Veatch believes we can conceive of cases in which personal identity may be lost but a death has not occurred. He interprets Green and Wikler as holding a functionalist, Lockean theory of personal identity in which psychological continuity of mental states accounts for personal identity over time. According to Veatch, Green and Wikler's theory would commit them to drawing the absurd conclusion that someone who has lost psychological continuity—for example, by suffering complete amnesia—has necessarily died. Veatch asks us to suppose that this human being who has suffered complete amnesia subsequently develops a new set of beliefs, memories, and other psychological characteristics that we associate with personhood. According to Veatch, even though we might regard such a being as a new person, it is counter-intuitive to say, as he believes Green and Wikler must say, that a death occurred in such a case. Thus, like Bernat, Culver, and Gert, Veatch assumes that *persons* are functional or qualitative specifications of human beings rather than substantive en-tities and concludes that such a view about persons and personal identity cannot pro-vide the proper grounding for a theory about death. Like Bernat and colleagues, Veatch believes human beings, not persons, are the kind of thing that dies. He ac-cepts what he says is the traditional Judeo-Christian concept of a human being as an essential union of mind and body. Since such a union may still exist even though someone suffers complete amnesia, the human being would still exist. A death has not occurred. An irreversible loss of consciousness, as in PermVS, however, would entail the destruction of the essential union of mind and body, and Veatch believes that the traditional Judeo-Christian concept of the human being thus requires ac-cepting a consciousness-related criterion of death. He regards individuals in PermVS as dead. The essential union of the mind and body has been destroyed.

Gervais has also criticized Green and Wikler's view, on similar grounds. She ar-gues that, as long as the biological substrate for consciousness remains intact despite the complete loss of memories, a death has not occurred. But she believes the same *person* continues to exist (Gervais 1986, 126). At this point, Gervais is invoking a sub-stantive concept of personhood and rejecting the functionalist view that she attrib-utes to Green and Wikler. In contrast to Veatch, Gervais treats persons as the kind of thing that can literally die. I believe she is correct in this and that Veatch errs in failing even to recognize a substantive concept of person. Gervais also reinterprets Veatch's argument in a way that essentially equates her substantive concept of per-son with his substantive concept of human being. Common to Gervais and Veatch is acceptance of the idea that what dies is a substantive entity that is essentially mind and body. Gervais calls such a being a "person," whereas Veatch refers to it as a "hu-man being." Gervais, like Veatch, also accepts a consciousness-related formulation of death that would treat individuals in PermVS as dead.

If Green and Wikler were indeed trying to defend a consciousness-related for-mulation of death on the basis of a functionalist theory of personal identity, then their argument would be subject to the criticisms of Veatch and Gervais. It is un-clear, however, that Green and Wikler are necessarily committed to the functional-ist view that Veatch and Gervais attribute to them. Green and Wikler consider a hypothetical case in which a brain may become "unwired" so completely "that the owner's entire complement of mental traits and capacities is permanently erased." In such a case of "brain zap," which would include complete amnesia, Green and Wikler believe that the person associated with those mental traits and capacities would no longer exist and should therefore be considered dead. This follows because "the ordinary causal processes which link events in a personal history involve more than spatiotemporal continuity of brain tissue. They also require continuity of certain brain *processes*, carried out through microstructural and microfunctional registrations in the brain tissue" (Green and Wikler 1980, 125–26). In the brain zap case, Green and Wikler may have assumed that the brain structures and processes that produce consciousness and other mental states are destroyed. They may not have considered Veatch's possibility of such a brain being reconstituted or rewired and subsequently producing consciousness, new experiences, and new memories.

The problem with evaluating the criticism leveled against Green and Wikler is that it is unclear what their view is. They believe the mere continuation of brain matter is insufficient for the continuation of personal identity. This is sensible. For example, we would not want to identify the person with his or her brain regardless of whether the brain matter was alive and functioning. Personal identity is not preserved by one's brain being preserved in formaldehyde. Minimally, the brain has to be functioning or, in Green and Wikler's terms, there must be "brain *processes*, carried out through microstructural and microfunctional registrations in the brain tissue" (126). It is unclear, however, whether Green and Wikler would view the continuation of the brain processes as sufficient for personal identity if psychological continuity in the form of memory connections were lost.

Veatch and Gervais interpret Green and Wikler as accepting a Lockean psychological continuity theory of personal identity. In Locke's view, an individual *a* at time t_1 is the same person as *b* at t_2 if and only if the mental states of *b* include memories of what *a* did; the substance that underlies the continuity of consciousness or memory relations, whether an immaterial soul, a human body, or a brain, is irrelevant to personal identity. Since psychological continuity, at least in the form of memory connections, is broken in the brain zap case, then, in Locke's view, the person who suffers the brain zap would have ceased to exist and the person with a new consciousness and memories after the brain zap would be a different person. Green and Wikler, however, link the continuity of consciousness to brain structures and processes in their account of personal identity, so it is unclear whether they are committed to the Lockean view.

Thus, while Green and Wikler would consider a person to have died if the structures and processes of the brain responsible for the person's consciousness, beliefs,

and memories were destroyed, what their view entails concerning Veatch's hypothetical case is uncertain. Whether the "unwiring" of the brain and "erasure" of the
memory involve the destruction of the brain is unclear. In Veatch's and Gervais's
hypothetical case, brain structures and processes are not completely destroyed, since
the brain is able to support consciousness, new thoughts, and new memories. The
continuous existence of brain structures and processes through the brain zap may
thus provide a basis for maintaining that the person continues to exist. Whether
Green and Wikler would accept this as a continuation of personal identity is uncertain, however, because it is unclear how Lockean their theory of personal identity is.
If they accept the Lockean psychological continuity theory, as Veatch and Gervais
interpret their doing, then Veatch's and Gervais's criticisms would apply. Since
Green and Wikler talk about the importance of brain structures and physical
processes, however, they seem to think the physical basis of psychological continuity is not irrelevant to personal identity, as a functionalist theory holds.

We should note that brain zap or complete memory loss is more hypothetical
than real. In actual cases of amnesia, even extreme cases, some memories and therefore some psychological continuity remain. This may provide a reason for thinking
that the same person is alive despite the amnesia, even in the functionalist theory of
personal identity. This same point would apply to the other cases Veatch is worried
about, such as dementia. Since some psychological connections remain, even in
cases of severe dementia, a functionalist could maintain that the same person persists through these changes. In addition, if the irreversible loss of all memories necessarily coincides with the irreversible destruction of the brain structures and
processes responsible for any form of consciousness, then there would be conceptual difficulty with the very intelligibility of the brain zap case.

Although Gervais presents the brain zap case as a counterexample to what she interprets Green and Wikler's view to be, she nowhere provides an argument for her
view that the same person continues to exist through brain zap. In other words, why
should the continuity of brain structures and processes that produce consciousness
and mental content be sufficient for the persistence of the same person, even in the
absence of memory connections between the mental states before and after the brain
zap? One could argue that the death of one substantive person has occurred and we
are witnessing the unusual generation of a new substantive person. Moreover, perhaps such a case forces us to reject the assumption that only one person may be connected with one human body during the life history of that body. I return to this
issue in the next chapter after presenting the substantive concept of personhood in
more detail. The substantive view that understands persons as constituted by, but not

identical to, human organisms enables us to maintain that a death has not occurred in the case of total amnesia and that the same person persists throughout.

PERSONS, PHILOSOPHY, AND CULTURE

Although the term *person* has various meanings and has been used in ordinary and technical language purportedly to refer to different kinds of things, this, of course, does not show that the term, in all or any of its uses, actually refers to anything and that one or more of the uses of the term cannot be dispensed with. There are plenty of instances in which terms used in ordinary as well as technical language were later shown to lack reference, such as *fairy*, *witch*, and *phlogiston*. In other words, although an analysis of ordinary language may reveal different uses of the term *person*, this does not show that all of those uses are sensible. It may turn out, upon reflection, that one or more of those uses are problematic because they lack reference, are useless in terms of explanation, or generate inconsistencies with other beliefs. Ultimately, the kinds of things that we admit into our ontology are determined by whether we have good empirical and theoretical reasons for their existence. Theory choice is, in turn, ultimately determined by considerations of explanatory power, testability, simplicity, consistency, and scope (Schick and Vaughn 2004).

In fact, much of the philosophical disagreement about persons and personal identity has focused on whether one or more of these concepts of person can be dispensed with entirely. For example, Derek Parfit (1986) rejects nonreductive, substantive theories of persons and the notion of personal *identity* that accompanies those theories. He also rejects the idea that persons are *identical to* physical organisms. Parfit accepts only a qualitative or functionalist view of persons and replaces the notion of personal identity with that of personal survival. What matters for Parfit in terms of personal survival is psychological continuity, regardless of the type of underlying causal basis of that continuity. Olson (1997), by contrast, rejects the idea that psychological continuity has anything to do with personal identity. He identifies the person with the biological organism and accordingly rejects both functionalist and substantive views that invoke notions of subjective experience or psychological continuity as essential to persons. Finally, those who argue for a nonreductive, substantive view of persons and personal identity reject the eliminative claims of these other theorists. In their view, a substantive theory best explains the wide range of our experience of persons and of what we wish to say about them.

When the discussion of personhood in the debate over abortion was perhaps at its height, Ruth Macklin (1983) concluded that we had reached an impasse of differences about the concept of personhood and that a continued focus on person-hood would be of little help in making progress or reaching any kind of consensus on abortion. Although Macklin provides a perceptive account of certain aspects of the disagreement over concepts of personhood and its role in bioethics, I think her conclusions were premature.

While I agree with Macklin that there will probably always be disagreement about the concept of person, I am generally skeptical about calling disagreement at any point "fundamental" or incapable of making progress toward consensus.[10] Fur-ther analysis often reveals how our beliefs are tied to other beliefs, and critical re-flection on those other beliefs may lead us to revise the beliefs that we thought were different in a "fundamental" or foundational sense. We sometimes find that what we initially considered to be a fundamental disagreement turns out to be a not so fun-damental disagreement or not even a disagreement at all. Indeed, because the con-cept of personhood is so central to our moral, metaphysical, and cultural systems of thought, it has a depth to it that we have only begun to explore. If Macklin is right that our concept of personhood is tied to other descriptive and prescriptive beliefs, we need to examine exactly what those beliefs are and whether they are consistent with how we use the term *person*.

As Daniel Callahan (1988) has pointed out, persons cannot be understood or de-fined by a single character or essential nature. Rather, our concept of person is com-plex and informed by biological, psychological, and cultural factors. Callahan quotes Ernest Becker, who observes, "In the human sciences man must be seen at all times in the total social-cultural-historical context, precisely because it is this that forms his 'self' or nature" (Callahan 1988, 47). This social-cultural-historical depth to the concept of person has been insufficiently explored, especially in the context of advances in life-sustaining technology that affect our understanding of when a person dies. Instead of uncritically accepting the medical or scientific paradigm of death, we need to explore our social-cultural-historical traditions and see how "brain death" fits with those traditions. On a broad public scale, such reflection has been done in Japan to a much greater extent than in other parts of the world (Lock 2002; LaFleur 2002, 2004; Morioka 2001). I believe that different concepts of personhood will prove to play a crucial role in explaining why people disagree about the defini-tion and criteria of death and that the moral of such a story is that we should accept pluralism in the definition and criteria of death. I hope, however, to identify some common beliefs within the Western philosophical tradition and across different social-cultural-historical traditions that can lead to a greater consensus on the defi-nition and criteria of death. For example, although philosophers in the Western tra-dition have disagreed over the sufficient conditions for personhood, there has been a great deal of agreement that the potential for consciousness is a minimal necessary condition. Such a consensus can provide the conceptual basis for accepting a consciousness-related formulation of death.

In addition, instead of examining how the social-cultural-historical context informs our notions of persons and personal identity, contemporary philosophers addressing issues of personhood, personal identity, and abortion have spent much more time considering conceptual puzzles about personal identity that ignore the social-cultural-historical context in which persons appear.[11] Although some theorists, such as G. H. Mead (1925, 1934), Jean-Paul Sartre ([1942] 1994; [1945] 1955; [1946] 1970), Ludwig Wittgenstein (1953), Clifford Geertz (1964, 1965, 1966), Rom Harré (1984, 1989), and Ken Gergen (1991a, 1991b), have emphasized the relational and cultural nature of persons, most contemporary debate over the criteria for personhood and personal identity in the philosophical literature has assumed that the criteria must be something internal to the person, such as internally related, psychological or bodily states. Much less attention has been paid to how external factors, such as an individual's relation to others or cultural factors, may determine the nature and identity of persons. An examination of such factors may lead to progress and greater consensus on the nature of persons and what it means for them to die. In fact, I shall argue that one of the main reasons for accepting the substantive view of persons as constituted by human organisms is that it allows for external factors to play an essential role in the identity and individuation of persons.

Furthermore, personhood is a dynamic concept that is subject to change in the light of new knowledge and possibilities. If there is some sense (and I think there is) to the existentialist idea that our nature is not fixed and that we can create, at least in part, who we are, then personhood and personal identity should be approached more as open-ended projects than as realities determined by factors independent of the choices we make. Thus, although examining our tradition is important for evaluating the new phenomena created by advances in medical technology, especially when it poses challenges to our concepts of life, death, and who we are, it is insufficient. We need to also ask what it is we want to become. We need to be open to the possibility that, just as there are new ways in which we can live, there may be new ways in which we can die.

In contrast to the eliminativist or reductionist strategies to consider persons as only human organisms or only functional specifications (modes), the three different uses of the term *person* have genuine reference. The references are to different kinds of things. Just as the word *bank* is not univocal and we are committed to the different kinds of things that we use this same word to refer to—a financial institution, the side of a river, for example—*person* can be used to refer to things associated with its different meanings. Moreover, just as it would be a mistake to insist that there are banks in the sense of financial institutions but no banks in the sense of the sides of rivers, it is a mistake to insist that there is nothing but human organisms or nothing but qualitative specifications of them. It is thus critical to identify the meaning of person that is intended when we say that a person has died. I agree with Bernat, Culver, and Gert that it would be a kind of category mistake or metaphor to attribute *death* to persons in the qualitative sense of the term. But it is not a mistake or metaphor to attribute *death* to persons in its species or substantive senses. Argument for commitment to the existence of persons in these two different senses must therefore be given.

CHAPTER FOUR

Persons as Substances

The current whole-brain neurological criterion for death specifies the cessation of all functions of the brain, including those of the brainstem. This criterion has come under attack from two sides: (1) by those who reject any brain-based criteria for death and argue for a return to the traditional circulatory and respiratory criteria and (2) by proponents of a consciousness-related formulation and criterion of death. Although these critics disagree over the definition and criteria of death, some of them share the same grounds for rejecting the current whole-brain criterion—that is, they reject the qualitative or functionalist view of personhood that underlies the biological paradigm. In the debate over the definition of death, it is thus critical to observe that proponents of the biological paradigm, particularly Bernat, Culver, and Gert, have selectively and without argument endorsed the qualitative or functionalist view of person to support their argument against (1) and (2). Since some proponents of (1) and (2) base their arguments on a substantive concept of personhood, those who adhere to the biological paradigm have never addressed the force of their objections. In short, because parties in the debate about the definition of death have been proposing definitions of death for different kinds of things, they have to a large extent been talking past each other. The fundamental issue of what it is that dies has not been engaged.

For example, one of the main reasons why Josef Seifert and D. Alan Shewmon have rejected any neurological criterion of death is that they reject Bernat, Culver, and Gert's qualitative or functionalist view of the person. Indeed, Seifert (1993, 182–83) and Shewmon (1997, 56) argue that acceptance of any neurological criterion for death, whole-brain or higher-brain, assumes a functionalist, or what they call an "actualist," view of personhood that is at odds with the substantive view of person found in the Catholic tradition. These critics also claim that such a view of personhood is "materially reductionist." I will have much more to say about Seifert's and Shewmon's views in chapter 6. At this point, I simply wish to note that Seifert and Shewmon are correct in their claim that the biological paradigm assumes a qualitative or functionalist view of the person and that such a view is at odds with the substantive view of personhood in the Catholic tradition.[1]

Shewmon and Seifert are mistaken, however, in thinking that any view that supports acceptance of a neurological criterion for determining death, including a consciousness-related criterion, assumes a qualitative or functionalist view of the person. Wallace (1995) and, in fact, Shewmon in his early work (1985) show that acceptance of a consciousness-related definition and neurological criterion of death is consistent with the substantive view of the person in the Catholic tradition. It is also consistent with a substantive view of personhood that can be found in the secular philosophical tradition.

In this chapter and the next, I examine and develop this secular, substantive view. I begin by focusing on the work of Peter Strawson and David Wiggins, two contemporary philosophers who view persons as substantive entities and not simply functional specifications of some more fundamental, underlying reality.[2] In their substantive view of person, it is neither a category mistake nor a metaphor to attribute death literally to persons. I also review and endorse Strawson's and Wiggins's reasons for rejecting the views that persons are immaterial souls or are identical to human organisms. Both philosophers treat *person* as a primitive concept in the sense that it cannot be analyzed or reduced to other, more fundamental concepts and that it gives a fundamental answer to the question of what exists.

I then consider the challenge to the substantive view posed by the case of total amnesia or brain zap. If persons and human organisms are both primitive but different kinds of substances, the case of total amnesia seems to generate a case of relative identity in which a (the individual before amnesia) is the same F (human organism) as b (the individual after amnesia), and a and b are both G (persons), but a is not the same G (person) as b. If identity is absolute, then there cannot be any genuine cases of relative identity.[3] By understanding the relation between the person and human organism as one of *constitution*, we avoid the threat of relative identity. Building on some of Wiggins's ideas, I argue that we should understand human persons as essentially psychological, moral, and cultural beings constituted by human organisms. The fundamental sortal concept by which we individuate and identify persons is a hybrid concept that combines the potential for subjectivity, other psychological activity, and moral standing with the type of organism that constitutes the person—for example, *human-person*. This view has several advantages. First, by treating persons as essentially but not identical to biological beings, we can incorporate the nomological grounding of natural kind concepts, such as human organism, into an account of person and, at the same time, treat persons as essentially psychological, moral, and cultural beings. This avoids the implausible view that *person* is strictly a natural kind concept and the unacceptable idea that *person* is simply a functional or artifactual concept susceptible to arbitrary stipulation. Second, the constitutive view provides the most consistent and plausible answers to questions raised by a range of problematic clinical and hypothetical cases, including whole-brain death, permanent vegetative state (PermVS), severe dementia, total amnesia, dissociative personality disorder, artificial persons, and thought experiments involving a purported replication of persons. Finally, the constitutive view recognizes that persons are partly determined by moral and cultural considerations. This allows for persons to be understood as open-ended projects, beings whose nature is not determined entirely by their biology but is, in part, a matter of personal and social construction.

STRAWSON'S VIEW

According to Peter Strawson, persons are individual entities to which predicates ascribing states of consciousness and predicates ascribing corporeal characteristics are equally applicable. He is critical of two types of views that would reject this claim and hold that "it is only a linguistic illusion that both kinds of predicate are properly ascribable to one and the same thing, that there is a common owner, or subject, of both types of predicate" (Strawson [1958] 1991, 105). The first view is Cartesian dualism, which holds that states of consciousness are ascribable only to immaterial minds or souls, to which corporeal predicates cannot be ascribed. The second view is what Strawson calls the "no-ownership" or "no-subject" doctrine of the self (106), which denies that states of consciousness belong to or are states of anything, "that it is a linguistic illusion that one ascribes one's states of consciousness at all, that there is any proper subject of these apparent descriptions" (105).[4] Both types of view, Strawson argues, cannot account for why one's states of consciousness are *ascribed* at all, to *any* subject.

Strawson is critical of a Cartesian view of the person that would ascribe states of consciousness to an immaterial, pure consciousness, ego, or mind, since this view makes it impossible to ascribe states of consciousness to others. If private experience is all that we have to go on in identifying the things to which states of consciousness are to be ascribed, then, "just for the very same reason as that for which there is, from one's own point of view, no question of telling that a private experience is one's own, there is also no question of telling that a private experience is another's. All private experience, all states of consciousness, will be mine, i.e., no one's" (108). Strawson's point is that "a necessary condition of states of consciousness being ascribed at all is that they should be ascribed to the *very same things* as certain corporeal characteristics, a certain physical situation, etc." (108). In other words, there is no sense to ascribing states of consciousness to oneself unless one knows how to ascribe states of consciousness to another, and this can be done only by using physical (behavioral) criteria in identifying others who are conscious.

Bernat, Culver, and Gert's qualitative or functionalist view is more akin to the "no-subject" view of the self, since they define personhood not in terms of a subject or entity but in terms of "certain abilities and qualities of awareness" (Culver and Gert 1982, 182–83; Bernat 2002, 330). Strawson is critical of such a view because it cannot coherently account for why one's states of consciousness are ascribed to a subject in a nontransferable sense, "in such a way that it is logically impossible that a particular state or experience in fact possessed by someone should have been possessed by someone else" (107). Presumably, Bernat, Culver, and Gert would say that, if the abilities and qualities of awareness that are definitive of personhood are possessed or had by anything, it would be not a Cartesian ego but the physical human body that stands in some unique causal relation to those abilities or qualities. They would construe this causal relationship as contingent, however: the abilities or experiences in question might have been causally dependent on a body other than the one on which they are actually dependent. The problem with this view, according to Strawson, is that it is incoherent. In claiming that the relationship is contingent and thereby denying any sense in which one's experiences are logically nontransferable, such theorists must rely on that very sense of nontransferable possession:

> It [the no-ownership view] is not coherent, in that one who holds it is forced to make use of that sense of possession of which he denies the existence in presenting his case for the denial. When he tries to state the contingent fact, which he thinks gives rise to the illusion of the "ego," he has to state it in some such form as "All *my* experiences are had$_1$ by (uniquely dependent on the state of) body B." For any attempt to eliminate the "my," or some other expression with a similar possessive force, would yield something that was not a contingent fact at all. The proposition that *all* experiences are causally dependent on the state of a single body B, for example, is just false. The theorist means to speak of all the experiences *had by a certain person* being contingently so dependent. And the theorist cannot consistently argue that "all the experiences of person P" *means*

the same thing as "all experiences contingently dependent on a certain body B"; for then his proposition would not be contingent, as his theory requires, but analytic. He must mean to be speaking of some class of experiences of the members of which it is in fact contingently true that they are all dependent on body B. And the defining characteristic of this class is in fact that they are "*my* experiences" or "the experiences *of* some person," where the sense of "possession" is the one he calls into question.

This internal incoherence is a serious matter when it is a question of denying what prima facie is the case: that is, that one does genuinely ascribe one's states of consciousness to something, viz., oneself, and that this kind of ascription is precisely such as the theorist finds unsatisfactory, i.e., is such that it does not seem to make sense to suggest, for example, that the identical pain which was in fact one's own might have been another's. We do not have to seek far in order to understand the place of this logically non-transferable kind of ownership in our general scheme of thought. For if we think of the requirements of identifying reference, in speech, to *particular* states of consciousness, or private experiences, we see that such particulars cannot be thus identifyingly referred to except as the states or experiences *of* some identified *person*. States or experiences, one might say, *owe* their identity as particulars to the identity of the person whose states or experiences they are. And from this it follows immediately that if they can be identified as particular states or experiences at all, they must be possessed or ascribable in just that way which the no-ownership theorist ridicules, i.e., in such a way that it is logically impossible that a particular state or experience in fact possessed by someone should have been possessed by anyone else. The requirements of identity rule out logical transferability of ownership. So the theorist could maintain his position only by denying that we could ever refer to particular states or experiences at all. And *this* position is ridiculous. (Strawson [1958] 1991, 106–7)

The upshot of Strawson's analysis is that the concept of person is "primitive" in the sense that it is not to be analyzed as a secondary kind of entity in relation to two primary kinds: a particular consciousness and a particular human body. He is critical of any straightforward identification of the person with the human body or some qualitative specification of the human body, since these views cannot coherently account for why *my* experiences are nontransferably *mine*. The implication of Strawson's concept of person for the debate over the definition of death is that it provides a conceptual basis for understanding the death of persons as the irreversible loss of consciousness or the breakdown of psychophysical integrity. Since persons are individual entities to which material and psychological predicates must equally apply, the loss of either set of predicates would entail the ceasing to exist (i.e., the death) of the person.

WIGGINS'S VIEW

David Wiggins is perhaps the leading contemporary proponent of a substantive view of personhood over a qualitative or functionalist view. Wiggins (1980, 171) holds that, although *person* is not synonymous with *human being*, we "feel" that these concepts are coextensive. He states, "on an understanding that is both psychologically and biologically replete of what it is for a man to have a life, the concepts *man* and *person* are sortally concordant and determine for anything falling in the extension of both a unitary principle of persistence—a principle that Locke himself admirably states in the words: '. . . the identity of the same *man* consists in nothing but a participation of the same continued life, by constantly fleeting particles of matter, in succession vitally united to the same organized body'" (161, n. 16, ellipsis in original).

Wiggins thus challenges Locke's view, as well as that of Bernat, Culver, and Gert, that questions concerning the identity of "man" should be distinguished from questions concerning the identity of "person." "However well one pushes the distinction between the concepts *man* and *person*," Wiggins writes, "this can hardly show that nothing falls under both concepts (under which is John Locke?), or that identity can be so relativized as to make the two identity questions independent of one another" (161, n. 16).

In Wiggins's account, a person is "an animal falling under the extension of a kind whose typical members perceive, feel, remember, imagine, desire, make projects, move themselves at will, speak, carry out projects, acquire a character as they age, are happy or miserable, are susceptible to concern for members of their own or like species, . . . [note carefully these and subsequent ellipses], conceive of themselves as perceiving, feeling, remembering, imagining, desiring, making projects, speaking . . . , have, and conceive of themselves as having, a past accessible in experience-memory and a future accessible in intention . . . , etc." (171, ellipses and bracketed note in original). He deliberately leaves his characterization of persons open for additional traits and makes no claim as to which particular traits are sufficient for being a person: "*person* is a concept whose defining marks are to be given in terms of a natural kind determinable, say *animal*, plus what may be called a functional or (as I shall prefer to say) systemic component" (171). In this "animal attribute" view, "a person is any animal that is such by its kind as to have the biological capacity to enjoy fully the psychological attributes enumerated" (172). His view thus treats persons as real, substantive entities and not just functional specifications of more fundamental, underlying realities.

Wiggins refers to the qualitative or functionalist view of the person as a "social constructivist" view (179). He is drawing a contrast between concepts that are artifactual and those that are nomologically grounded. Artifactual concepts can be freely reconceptualized and reinterpreted at any time, whereas concepts that are nomologically grounded, such as natural kind concepts, are a matter for discovery. Following Putnam and Leibniz, the view of natural kinds to which Wiggins is appealing is one that "stands or falls with the existence of lawlike principles that will collect together the actual extension of the kind around an arbitrarily good specimen of it; and . . . these lawlike principles will also determine the characteristic development and typical history of members of this extension (or at least the limits of any possible development or history of such individuals)" (169–70).

According to Wiggins, *person* is "similar" or "akin" to a natural kind concept, such as human being (170).[5] However, *person* is not a natural kind concept, because it contains a psychological component that is "supervenient" on the notion of physical nature associated with the natural kind *human being*. This supervenient relationship between the person and the human being allows for the dependency of human persons on human animals (persons are not simply artifactual constructions), but persons are not reducible or identical to human animals (183, n. 40). Thus, the interdependence of the concepts *person* and *human being*—that is, some things "falling under" both concepts—and an understanding that is "both psychologically and biologically replete of what it is for a man to have a life" do not require that the concept of person and human animal are sortally concordant.[6] Instead, the psychological and biological factors of what it is for a man to be alive and persist and what it is for a person to be alive and persist may differ, and, therefore, the concepts *man* and *person* are not necessarily either sortally concordant or coextensive. Wiggins thus does not *identify* the person with the human being but construes persons as naturally *supervening* on human beings.

It is also clear that Wiggins does not accept a "species meaning" of persons in the way that, for example, Fred Feldman does. Wiggins argues directly against a simple, bodily continuity criterion of personal identity when he writes that "bodily continuity is not enough without life" (Wiggins 1980, 162). As Feldman (1992) maintains, if persons are identical to their bodies, persons who have died but whose bodies are preserved would have to be counted among present persons. Wiggins considers the view of Bernard Williams that we should simply say that the deceased are dead persons, but he argues, "It may be said that we can and do distinguish between the corpse of a man freshly dead—he is still here but dead—and his earthly remains. When ashes (say) are all that is left, then he is no longer there, it may be suggested. But the whole distinction which is relied on is parasitic upon the point of distinguishing between life and death. Mere material continuity is not sufficient. And if life or its absence gives the *point* of these distinctions, then the *principal* distinction is between being alive and being dead, and the best overall view will make existence or non-existence depend upon the principal distinction" (Wiggins 1980, 162, n. 17). According to Wiggins, Aunt Ethel, the person, has ceased to exist upon her death. What gets interred is not a person but the bodily remains of one.

Although Wiggins clearly rejects the species meaning of person, his response is problematic. Williams and Feldman could employ Wiggins's own definition of a person to counter his response. Why, they might ask, can't we identify, say, the well-preserved pharaoh as an animal that, in Wiggins's own words, "is such *by its kind* as to have the biological capacity to enjoy fully the psychological attributes enumerated"? (Wiggins 1980, 172, emphasis added). Certainly, the mummified pharaoh belongs to this kind of animal rather than to a kind of animal that lacks psychological capacities or potentials. That the pharaoh as a member of the human species may lack the biological capacity for life or psychological attributes should not matter if Wiggins wishes to define persons by their membership in a kind rather than in terms of whether the individual member of the kind has the capacity or potential for the functions that we associate with being a person.

In response to this objection, Wiggins could maintain that being alive is essential to being a member of certain natural kinds, so the human corpse is no longer a natural kind of thing—that is, an animal. This would be consistent with his "animal attribute" view of person: that being an animal is necessary for being a person. In this view, the body of Aunt Ethel is not a person because it is not even an animal. This strategy would amount to a revision of the species meaning of person, since membership in the kind *Homo sapiens* would require being alive. Thus, in challenging Williams and Feldman, Wiggins would invoke an aspect of the functional or systemic component that he claims is necessary for the existence of human beings: human beings must be alive. Simply being a specimen of the biological species *Homo sapiens* is insufficient for being a human *being*. Moreover, because being an animal is necessary for being a person, the pharaoh cannot be a person. This view, of course, accords with Wiggins's later claim that artifacts such as robots and automata, in contrast to higher-order animals such as dolphins and apes, cannot possibly be persons. He asserts that, "to have genuine feeling or purposes or concerns, a thing must *at least* be an animal" (175).

Thus, according to Wiggins, our judgment that the pharaohs do not exist and are not to be counted among present persons should be based on the distinction between life and death and the fact that the pharaohs are dead. Life is a minimal, necessary condition for being a person. Wiggins's revised "species meaning" of person would also allow for the possibility of holding that membership in the species is sufficient for personhood, which is one way of interpreting the passage quoted above in which he states that "a person is any animal that is such by its kind as to have the biological capacity to enjoy fully the psychological attributes enumerated" (172). I do not think, however, that Wiggins would endorse this view, for several reasons. His point is not that every human being is a person but the more modest one that human beings, as opposed to, say, snails, are the kind of thing that can be persons.

First, although Wiggins fixes the extension of the concept of person by reference to paradigmatic examples of persons, such as you and I, he is reticent about specifying which aspects of his neo-Lockean activity-grounded principle for the identity and individuation of person are necessary and sufficient for being a person. Instead, he is committed to two minimal, necessary conditions of person: that persons must be living animals and that they satisfy to some degree the psychological, systemic component. To regard every living human being as a person would involve commitment to sufficient conditions for personhood that are too restrictive, a commitment that Wiggins is not prepared to make: "being a man or being a human being is the only thing that we can make stand proxy for what it is to be a person" (Wiggins 1980, 174). He believes, however, that "although we can begin a list of important attributes of people and see how some faculties are nested in others, we have no firm grasp at all of how to fill in the dots in the proposed specification of what a person is" (173). His point is that we are in the process of discovering the nature of persons and that, at this point in our investigation, any human being may be assumed to be a person. This does not rule out the possibility that, as our inquiry proceeds, some of the humans that we have assumed to be persons will turn out not to be persons or that some humans sustained in novel, artificial ways are not persons. By analogy, in the process of investigating the nature of water, we may have relied on samples of liquids that in the end prove not to be water. Thus, just as it would have been premature to say that any clear liquid must be water before discovering the nature of water, so, too, it would be premature to say that any human being is a person.

Second, although Wiggins states that "persons are a class of organism," his remarks about persons supervening on human organisms suggest that persons are not reducible or identical to human organisms. Part of the difficulty in interpreting Wiggins is that he does not offer a developed account of the notion of supervenience that he is relying on. He cites Donald Davidson's use of the concept of supervenience in understanding the relation between the mental and the physical and G. E. Moore's use of the concept to reject ethical naturalism—the view that good is reducible by predicates standing for the physical or natural properties of things or by some complex of such predicates (Wiggins 1980, 182–83).[7] Davidson and Moore understand supervenience as a relation of dependency but nonreducibility. The supervenient entities, whether they are mental states (Davidson), values (Moore), or persons

(Wiggins), are dependent on physical states or natures but are not reducible to them. This means there are no strict deterministic laws governing how the supervening properties, states, or entities can be explained or predicted. Consequently, applied to Wiggins's view, the individuation and identity of the human being (the supervenience base) does not necessarily entail the individuation and identity of a person (the supervening entity).

Third, there is a problem of consistency if Wiggins wishes to maintain that membership in the living species *Homo sapiens* is sufficient for being a person. In defining personhood, Wiggins invokes what he calls a "neo-Lockean activity-grounded principle of individuation for persons" (Wiggins 1980, 164). Persons are not just living animals but must satisfy a systemic component that may include the capacity to "perceive, feel, imagine, desire, make projects" (171). As mentioned above, Wiggins believes we may not be able to specify which particular elements of the psychological, systemic component may be necessary or sufficient for a member of the natural kind *human being* to count as a person. It is clear that, for Wiggins, at least some of these elements must be present or potentially present. Indeed, he considers the possibility that some other higher-order animals, such as dolphins and apes, may be persons, precisely because these other animals may satisfy the systemic component. Again, the defining marks of the concept *person* are animality *plus* the psychological, systemic component.

We can ask how Wiggins would explain cases in which there is a living human body—for example, the anencephalic or individual in PermVS—but no sign of the systemic component (Wiggins's neo-Lockean activity principle) necessary for that living human body to count as a person. In these cases, the neurophysiological basis of *any* of the psychological functions that typical persons manifest is nonexistent. Though anencephalics and individuals in PermVS may be living members of the biological species human being, they lack the capacity and potential for any of the above psychological functions and therefore, on Wiggins's account, are not persons. Thus, since the life of a person does not necessarily correspond to the life of a human body, Wiggins must recognize a distinction between the existence and persistence conditions of human beings and of persons and therefore reject even a revised "species meaning."

Wiggins is concerned that this distinction between the concepts *person* and *human being* would threaten his general view of identity and individuation; in particular, the distinction would generate a case of relative identity (R) in which *a* is the same F as *b*, and *a* is also a G, but *a* is not the same G as *b*. Take the case of an individual, such as Nancy Cruzan, who suffers severe anoxia as a result of injuries sustained in an automobile accident and thereafter persists in a permanent vegetative state. Given the distinction between a person and a human being, we could say that Cruzan at t_1, before her accident, is the same human being as Cruzan at t_2, two years after her accident, and that Cruzan at t_1 is also a person, but that Cruzan at t_1 is not the same person as Cruzan at t_2. Since, as Wiggins believes, identity is absolute, there cannot be any genuine cases of relative identity. The absoluteness of identity requires that if a is the same F as b, and a is also G, then a is the same G as b. Wiggins's concern about violating this principle would thus lead him to claim that Cruzan is the same human organism and person throughout. Despite Wiggins's worry, I believe this is not a genuine case of relative identity and that the distinction is therefore innocuous to the absoluteness of identity. If the relationship between the person and the human being is one of "supervenience" or "constitution," as Wiggins suggests, then this case can be explained along the lines that Wiggins (1980, 30–35) offers in his discussion of "type-(4)" purported cases of relative identity, where he employs the notion of the constitutive sense of *is*.

The challenge that the case of PermVS poses to our concepts of human being and person is similar to that posed by the case of total amnesia or "brain zap," considered in chapter 3. For, if we interpret a case of total amnesia as one in which "the man who begins life anew after total amnesia is the same organism or animal as, but a different person from, the man who lost his memory"(176), then we might be thought to have a genuine case of relative identity. Indeed, because Wiggins believes such an interpretation of total amnesia would violate the absoluteness of identity, he rejects it. He believes the same human being and person persist through total amnesia. Thus, if Smith at t_1, before amnesia, is the same human organism as Smith at t_{10}, after the onset of amnesia, and Smith at t_1 is also a person, then Smith at t_1 must be the same person as Smith at t_{10}.

Finally, cases of "multiple personality" or "dissociative personality disorder" may be thought to challenge the absoluteness of identity in a similar way. If this phenomenon genuinely involves two or more substantive persons in one body, each taking control of the body at different times, then the following case of relative identity would arise: Dr. Jekyll could be the same human being as Mr. Hyde, and Dr. Jekyll would also be a person, but Dr. Jekyll would not be the same person as Mr. Hyde.

To respond to the challenge that these cases, involving a distinction between the human organism and person, would threaten the absoluteness of identity, two options are available. First, *person* may be interpreted as a phased sortal—that is, as a concept that may apply during a certain period of the life history of an individual identified under some substance concept (Wiggins 1980, 24–27). For example, as noted in chapter 2, caterpillar and butterfly are phased sortals of the substance sortal lepidoptera. *Lepidoptera* applies throughout the life history of individuals identified under the concept, whereas *caterpillar* and *butterfly* apply only at certain times or phases of the substance identified under the concept *lepidoptera*. *Boy, adult, banker, conscript* are other common examples of phased sortals. Thus, if person is a phase of the human organism, *human organism* would apply throughout the life history of the individuals identified by the concept, whereas *person* would apply only during a certain phase, such as when the human organism has the capacity for consciousness and other mental abilities. Cruzan would thus have been in a person phase as long as she retained the capacity for consciousness. Indeed, the functionalist or qualitative view of persons treats person as a phase of the substantial kind *human organism*. Substance concepts, in contrast to phased sortal concepts, provide the most fundamental answers to the question "what is x?" Thus, interpreting person as a phase of some more fundamental underlying substance (e.g., human organism) would entail giving up the idea that, in our ontology, persons are primitive substances. Although this interpretation would dispense with the purported cases of relative identity,[8] Strawson has given good reasons for why *person* must be treated as a primitive, substantive concept and not as a qualification or phase of some other primitive, substantive concept. I will give additional reasons for rejecting the phased sortal interpretation in chapter 7, where I examine more fully the qualitative or functionalist view of person.

The second way to respond to the problem of how the distinction between persons and human organisms may generate a case of relative identity is to construe the relation between the person and human organism as one of constitution. This constitutive interpretation enables us to retain the idea that persons are primitive substantive entities and to consistently interpret cases of total amnesia, multiple personality, and PermVS without violating the absoluteness of identity. It also provides the basis for treating the person as a kind of thing that dies.

CHAPTER FIVE

The Constitutive View of Persons

In an earlier work (Lizza 1991), I argued that the relation between the person and the human organism should be understood as one of constitution.[1] Following Tyler Burge's discussion (1975) of how the notion of constitution captures the relation between ordinary objects, such as balls and tables, and the kind of stuff they are made of, such as gold or wood, I suggested that constitution should not be restricted to the relation between the references of count nouns and mass terms. The notion of constitution is also helpful in other contexts to understand the relation between two kinds of things that we commonly admit into our ontology but that coincide in their spatiotemporal location. I also argued that subjectivity is essential to persons and that persons and personal identity are determined, in part, by moral and cultural factors.

More recently, Lynne Rudder Baker (2000) developed much more fully the view that persons are constituted by human beings.[2] She, too, treats subjectivity as essential to persons and has shown how relational factors play a role in their constitution. Like Joseph Margolis (1984), Baker points out that some relational properties of persons and other objects, such as works of art, are intentional: they have essential properties that require propositional attitudes. Thus, Michelangelo's *David* could not exist except in relation to an art world. Similarly, persons cannot exist independent of their having and being related to beings with propositional attitudes. While not all constituted things have intentional properties—for example, genes are constituted by DNA molecules but existed before there were propositional attitudes—others, such as persons and works of art, are dependent on their relation to beings with intentionality (Baker 2000, ch. 2). This last factor provides the conceptual space to do justice to the role of social and cultural factors in fixing the boundaries of our concept of person, factors that theorists such as Mead, Sartre, Geertz, and Harré have emphasized in their work.

In this chapter, I begin by showing how the constitutive interpretation can be used to respond to the threat of relative identity posed by cases of total amnesia, dissociative personality disorder, and permanent vegetative state (PermVS). The constitutive interpretation allows, in principle, for the possibility that total amnesia and dissociative personality disorder may involve two or more persons being constituted by the same human organism during its life history. It also allows for the possibility that, with PermVS, a human organism can constitute a person at one time in its life history but not at another. In short, this interpretation allows for the conditions for the individuation and identity of persons to diverge from those of the human organism without violating the absoluteness of identity. The constitutive interpretation, however, does not necessitate our interpreting these cases in the way described. In fact, some further considerations about how persons are constituted by human bodies should lead us to reject the possibility of a human organism constituting more than one person during its life history. These same considerations support the interpretation that human persons who have lost the brain functions necessary for consciousness have died, even if the human organism continues to exist.

Another problem addressed here is whether the constitutive interpretation allows for the possibility that a person constituted by a human organism at one time could be constituted at some later time by a different organism (human or of another species) or by artificial, bionic matter. This problem is particularly interesting in the context of determining death. For if it were possible to gradually replace human organic parts with bionic ones without destroying subjectivity and psychological continuity, we might have a new way to beat the reaper and achieve immortality. But, as I argue in this chapter, the same considerations that lead us to reject the possibility that more than one substantive person can be constituted by a single human organism during its life history should lead us to reject this possibility as well.

THE CONSTITUTIVE VIEW

In *Sameness and Substance*, David Wiggins (1980) critiques the continuity criterion of personal identity. He introduces the idea that the *is* in statements such as "Caesar is that human being or that human body" should be understood not as the *is* of identity but as the *is* of constitution. He claims, "A person is material in the sense of being essentially constituted by matter; but in some strict and different sense of 'material,' viz. being definable or properly describable in terms of the concepts of the sciences of matter (physics, chemistry, and biology even) person is not a material concept" (Wiggins 1980, 164). His claim is that an entity can be counted and individuated as a person only if it satisfies a neo-Lockean activity-grounded principle. This continuity principle, he argues, "defines a material entity in the 'matter-constituted' sense of 'material,' while leaving it possible for the concept person to be both primitive relative to the concepts that pull their weight in the sciences of matter and primitive relative to the concept human body. If we understand what a living person or animal is, then we may define the body of one as that which realizes or constitutes it while alive and will be left over when, succumbing to entropy, it dies" (164).

It is puzzling that, in the very next paragraph, he remarks that the way in which persons transcend bodies is "reminiscent in some ways of the constitutive 'is' introduced in Chapter One" (164). Why should there be any significant difference between how the constitutive *is* functions in an explanation of the relation between a person and a human body and that of the relation between, say, a jug and a collection of material bits from which it is constituted? As far as the constitutive *is* is concerned, it is irrelevant whether the relation is between animate or inanimate objects.

As noted in chapter 4, Wiggins is concerned about the possibility of a human body constituting more than one person during its life span, but he accepts this kind of possibility in the case of inanimate objects—for example, when someone uses the material bits of a broken jug to make a coffee pot. But why should Wiggins be concerned about a human body constituting more than one person over its life span? If the *is* in "Dr. Jekyll is that human being" or "Dr. Jekyll is a human being" is the constitutive *is* and not the *is* of identity, then the possibility of two or more persons sharing one body, each taking his or her turn to control it, does not represent a case of relative identity. Moreover, the possibility of Smith at t_1, before amnesia, being a different person from Smith at t_2, after onset of amnesia, would not represent a case of relative identity. The reasons why these cases do not entail relative identity are given by Wiggins himself in his discussion of purported "type-(4)" cases of relative identity.

Consider the following two alleged examples of type-(4) relative identity:

(α)   I might say to someone "that heap of fragments there is the jug you saw the last time you came to this house." They could not be *the same jug* but they might be *the same collection of material bits*.

(β)   The visitor might be a person of tiresome ingenuity and cement the pieces of the jug together to make not a jug but, say, a coffee pot of a quite different shape from the original jug's. It might then be said that "the jug is the coffee pot" is true with covering-concept *same collection of material bits* and false with covering-concept *same utensil*. (Wiggins 1980, 27–28)

Wiggins points out that "(α) and (β) hang together. For if the jug is the same collection of bits as the heap of fragments and the heap of fragments is the same collection of bits as the coffee pot, then, by transitivity, the jug must be the same collection of bits as the coffee pot. Either both or neither, then, is a true identity-statement. The difficulty is that if the jug is the same collection of material parts, bits of china clay, as the coffee pot, that is if they are one and the same collection of china-bits, then their life-histories and durations must be the same. But the coffee pot *will* be fabricated or assembled at t_3 by my ingenious friend and exist only from then on. The jug won't then exist any more." He asserts that, to have the sort of type-(4) relative identity statement that the relativist requires, "the '*is*' in 'is the same collection of china-bits' of (α) and (β) must mean '=' and we must take *collection of china-bits* as a straightforward covering-concept" (30). Given the life-history principle that if a (e.g., jug) and b (e.g., collection of china bits) are identical, then they must have the same life history, Wiggins argues as follows:

> Suppose I destroy the jug. Do I then destroy the collection? Either I do or I don't. If I do then both (α) and (β) fail of truth with covering concept *collection of china-bits* and fail as type-(4) examples. If I don't thus destroy the collection then it cannot be true of the jug that it *predicatively* is a collection of china-bits. But nevertheless it is *true* that the jug is a collection of china-bits. That is to say that it is china-clay. Therefore it must be true but not straightforwardly *predicatively* true. I suggest that it is true in the sense that the jug is *made of* china-clay or *constituted of* china-bits. *This* is what is predicatively true of the jug. (31)

An analogous argument can deal with a case of multiple persons or personality that is purported to be an example of type-(4) relative identity: "(κ) Dr. Jekyll and Mr. Hyde were the *same man* but not the *same person* or *personality*" (29). Wiggins considers (κ) to be an alleged example of type-(5) relative identity and accordingly disposes of (κ) as a case of ambiguous reference in which "'Dr. Jekyll' and 'Mr. Hyde' have . . . to be read twice over in (κ) to make it come out true, first as standing each for a man (this individual is the same man as that individual), the second time as standing for a certain kind of character or personality. (These personalities, not these men, are different.) But this ruins the prospects of seeing it as a case of R; and the example really represents an implausible attempt to postulate philosophically defined schizophrenia without going the whole way and postulating two men

sharing one body, each taking his turn to control it" (37). The difficulty raised, however, is arguably of type-(4) and can be handled as such. For to consider (κ) as type-
(4), we need only take seriously the claim that it represents a case of two persons
sharing one body, each taking his turn to control it.

If we understand (κ) as entailing two persons sharing one body, however, the
difficulty is similar to that encountered in (α) and (β). If Jekyll is the same human
being (man or body) as Hyde—if they share one and the same human being or
body—then their life histories and durations must be the same. But Hyde did things
at Tilbury Docks that Jekyll did not do. Therefore, Jekyll did not exist at Tilbury
Docks. But by understanding the *is* in "Dr. Jekyll is the same man as Mr. Hyde" as
a constitutive *is*, we can paraphrase Wiggins's argument in his discussion of (α) and
(β) to resolve the difficulty. Thus, if *a* (Jekyll) and *b* (a particular human being or
body) are identical, then they must have the same life history. Now suppose I destroy
Jekyll by destroying his capacity to enjoy some or all of the psychological attributes
associated with the concept *person*. (Suppose I can destroy Jekyll's systemic component without destroying the biological capacity of Hyde or any other person to enjoy psychological functions associated with the concept *person*.) Now, do I thus destroy the man or human body with which Jekyll is alleged to be identical? Either I
do or I don't. If I do, then (κ) fails of truth with the covering-concept *man* and fails
as a type-(4) example. If I do not, then it could not be true of Jekyll that he *predicatively* is a human being. Nevertheless, it is *true* that Jekyll is a human being; that is
to say, Jekyll is human. Therefore, it must be true in the sense that Jekyll is *made of*
human matter or *constituted by* a living human body. *This* is what is predicatively
true of Jekyll.

Note that if person and human being did have the same principle of individuation, (κ) would still not be a genuine example of R. For in this case Jekyll would not
be the same human being as Hyde. Because Jekyll and Hyde have different life histories and because we have no plausible alternative to Leibniz's law, *human being*
could not be a proper covering-concept for persons in the same way that *collection
of china-bits* could not be a proper covering-concept for artifacts.

The upshot of this analysis is that it enables us to respect the absoluteness of identity and at the same time appraise total amnesia ("brain zap") and dissociative personality disorder as cases in which we have the same human organism but different
persons. Similarly, we can appraise the case of PermVS as one in which the human
being or organism persists, even though the person no longer does. While such
interpretations are consistent with the absoluteness of identity, we should not interpret all of these cases in this way. In fact, as I argue below, these interpretations of
total amnesia and dissociative personality disorder are incorrect. In the case of total

amnesia, the same substantive person persists despite the loss of memories. In the case of multiple personality, or the descriptively better "dissociative personality disorder," the different "persons" or "personalities" are persons or personalities in the qualitative sense of the term, not the substantive sense. Thus, dissociative personality disorder does not represent a case of more than one substantive person being constituted by a single human being over the course of that human being's life history. However, the cases of total amnesia and dissociative personality disorder differ from the cases of PermVS and whole-brain death in a significant way. Since the neurophysiological basis for subjectivity and all psychological functions is destroyed in PermVS and whole-brain death, the human organism that constituted the person can no longer constitute one. The person has thus died, even though the human organism or some kind of living organism may continue to exist.

HUMAN-PERSONS

My reasons for rejecting the interpretation that, in cases of total amnesia and dissociative personality disorder, there may be more than one substantive person constituted synchronically or diachronically by a human organism are based on several considerations. First, although the constitutive relation itself allows, in principle, for more than one thing to be constituted by the same matter over time (e.g., the jug may be constituted by the same collection of material bits as the coffee pot), there is a great deal more flexibility of manipulation when inanimate matter constitutes more than one kind of inanimate thing than when a natural kind of living thing (e.g., a human organism) constitutes another kind of living thing (e.g., a person). Here, the distinction between natural kinds and artifacts (i.e., between concepts that are nomologically grounded and those that are not) is relevant.

Following Wiggins's treatment of *person* as "akin" to a natural kind concept, when a natural kind constitutes another kind, the nomological grounding of the natural kind restricts the possibilities for the kind of thing that it constitutes. For example, because human beings are not the kind of thing that can undergo amoeba-like splitting, persons constituted by human beings are not the kind of thing that can undergo amoeba-like splitting. Thus, although the laws that govern the extension of the concept *human organism* do not completely determine the extension of the concept *person*, they are relevant to determining the conditions for the individuation and identity of persons. The relation of constitution introduces something more than bodily and psychological continuity in considering issues of personal identity. It is an additional fact about persons that may be appealed to when evaluating problematic cases at the beginning and end of a person's life.

To see how the individuation and identity of persons are dependent on the individuation and identity of human beings, it may be helpful to review Wiggins's general line of argument in *Sameness and Substance*. In summary, he claims the following:

1. Everything that exists is a *this such*—that is, it is dependent on a sortal concept for its individuation (15).

2. Natural kind concepts are sortal concepts that are nomologically grounded; that is, there are true lawlike principles in nature for the actual extension of a natural kind predicate, which are collected together around the focus of an actual specimen (84).[3]

3. If this lawlikeness is a requirement for the sense of the natural kind predicate, "then it is a condition of the very existence of *f*s [objects falling under the sortal concept *f*], so defined, that certain lawlike sentences should hold true" (84).

4. The lawlike sentences "must determine directly or indirectly, in ways that we can uncover by empirical discovery, the characteristic development, the typical history, and the limits of any possible development or history of any compliant of *f*" (84).

5. ". . . a particular continuant *x* belongs to a natural kind, or is a natural thing, if and only if *x* has a principle of activity corresponding to the nomological basis of that or those extension-involving sortal identifications which answer truly the question 'what is *x*'" (89). Here, Wiggins draws a distinction between nature and artifact to mark the distinction between concepts that are nomologically founded and those that are not (175, n. 30). Wiggins claims that the concept *person*, if not coextensive with the natural kind concepts *man* and *human being*, is at least akin to a natural kind concept. He writes, "Persons are a class of organisms, and they are identified under concepts that are nomologically conditioned. Whatever else they may be, they are things in nature. Artifacts, on the other hand, which are not in and of nature but often beneficially displace nature, are not identified under concepts that are nomologically conditioned" (187).

6. Sentience, desire, belief, motion, memory, and various other elements are involved in the particular mode of activity that marks the extension of the concept of person (160).

As noted in chapter 4, while Wiggins holds that a certain mode of activity is essential to the individuation of persons, it is unclear just what that activity consists of. He does suggest that there is something sensible in the Lockean notion that "a person is an object essentially aware of its progress and persistence through time, and peculiar among all other kinds of things by virtue of the fact that its present being is always under the cognitive and affective influence of its experiential memory of what it was in the past" (Wiggins 1980, 150). He formulates the "*C-relation" as an amendment to Locke's requirement of continuity of consciousness for personal identity over time. For Wiggins, the C-relation represents the strong continuity of consciousness or memory relation that Locke insisted obtains between person P_{tj} and person Q_{tk}, if P and Q are identical (Wiggins 1980, 154, n. 8; P [or Q] designates a definite description of a continuing person, not of a time slice, and subscripts tj and tk index the time at which the definite description applies to the continuing person).

According to Wiggins, Locke's C-relation states that, "for some sufficiency of things actually done, witnessed, experienced . . . at any time by P_{tj}, Q_{tk} should later have sufficient real or apparent recollection of then doing, witnessing, experiencing them" (154). Locke's identity condition thus makes the persistence of a person P depend only upon P's being related at each successive phase of his biography in this C-relation to P at each previous phase. "C itself," Wiggins points out, "is a non-transitive relation" (155).

To counter Joseph Butler's charge that Locke's continuity of consciousness criterion entails the absurd conclusion that "a person has not existed a single moment, not done one action, but what he can remember; indeed none but what he reflects upon" (Butler [1736] 1975, 100), Wiggins offers the *C-relation, the ancestral of the C-relation, which is "the weaker and transitive relation of x being either C-related to y or C-related to some z which is C-related to y or . . ." (Wiggins 1980, 155). Wiggins calls this simply co-consciousness and states that it provides us with a "general neo-Lockean identity condition: I_p: P is the same person as Q if and only if $(Q)^*C(P)$" (155). Wiggins goes on to say that, while $(Q)^*C(P)$ avoids the defects of circularity, it has defects that relate to "(i) the formal inadequacy of $(x)^*C(y)$ to define an equivalence relation like identity, and (ii) the need to fortify *C in order to secure what is actually intended by the continuity of consciousness requirements" (155).

Defect (i) arises because *C is not necessarily transitive and symmetrical—that is, not necessarily a one-one relation—and hence cannot be sufficient for identity. For nothing Wiggins has said has yet ruled out the possibility of a stream of consciousness dividing at some point and flowing into a delta of two consciousnesses that are separate thereafter. Thus, if it is conceivable that $(Q_{t3})^*C(P_{t1})$ and $(R_{t3})^*C(P_{t1})$, the symmetry of the *C relation is threatened and, therewith, the possibility of its serving as a characterization of personal identity. Wiggins considers, however, the possibility that for *persons* properly understood, such a division is not conceivable. "But," writes Wiggins, "that will not necessarily invalidate the objection. For we may find that, if such a division is in fact impossible, then this impossibility derives *from the conceptual requirements on the individuation of persons:* in which case the impossibility should be deducible from the right hand side of I_p or the *C requirement. But it is not so deducible. Therefore, I_p is at very best an inadequate elucidation of the identity of persons. Either then I_p is actually wrong, or else I_p is inadequate" (158, emphasis added).

Defect (ii) arises because *C offers no plausible account of error and hence cannot designate the kind of mental continuity demanded by Locke. Wiggins explains.

> Suppose that at t_3 I think that I vividly remember locking the back door, though the fact is that some well disposed neighbor slipped the latch (at t_2) after I had gone off without locking up. Then, unless we are already possessed of a criterion of identity or something else to refute the memory claim itself, we seem to have:
>
> > (Wiggins who at t_3 imagines he remembers locking the door)*C(person who slipped the latch at t_2).
>
> This is bad enough, but suppose that later at t_4 I begin to doubt that I locked the door, remembering that at t_3 I had supposed that I vividly remembered doing so. Then it may be held
>
> > (Wiggins who doubts at t_4 that he locked the door)*C(Wiggins who thought at t_3 he remembered locking the door).
>
> But then whether I like it or not, *C must by the intended transitivity and symmetry hold (even as I doubt) between me and the man or woman who locked the back door. But here I don't have even what Locke intended by continuity of consciousness with the person who locked it. And insisting on the "sufficiency of things" hedge that we introduced at the beginning of section 3 into the definition of C and *C, or stiffening the subjective requirements on remembering locking the door (the amplitude, stability, richness, etc., of the inner representation), will scarcely alter the position. The troublesome example itself could always be correspondingly enriched. (158)

In short, it seems that we need some criterion independent of memory claims—that is, bodily continuity—to check whether memory claims are true. This implies not that bodily continuity is sufficient for personal identity but that it may be a necessary condition.

Wiggins's correct response to defect (ii) is that the defect shows only that memory by itself is not sufficient for determining answers to the identity questions. It does not show that memory does not contribute or, with other considerations of what it means for persons to be alive and leading a life, that memory is not crucial to our choice of a continuity principle for persons. He concludes that Locke's definition of personal identity "does not oblige us to say that memory determines identity questions autonomously; only that it contributes and, in conjunction with other considerations, is crucially relevant to our choice of a continuity principle for determining the biographies of persons. What the objection really had to confront was a thesis about memory as part and parcel with other vital functions and faculties characteristic of persons. But against this thesis it simply begs the question" (162).

Following Wiggins, we should conclude that *C may be an important but not sufficient condition for the continuity principle of persons. We should note further, however, that, in Wiggins's account, memory is not even a necessary condition of personal identity. Since he regards *person, man,* and *human being* as sortally concordant concepts and even coextensive, he believes that a complete loss of memory (a lack of the *C-relation) should not affect our judgment of a person's identity over time. He asserts that there are, at most, four ways of appraising a case of total amnesia:

(1)   We may hold that it voids any application of the concept of person. But in practice, when people do lose their memory, we never adopt this view.

(2)   We may attempt to do honour to *C by deciding that the man who begins life anew after total amnesia is the same organism or animal as, but a different person from, the man who lost his memory. This is a tempting but incoherent decision . . . If y is the same animal as x, and y is a person, then y is the person that x was. But then y is the same person as x.

(3)   We may decide to say that, because y has no hope of playing x's role, y is a different person from x, and so (by Leibnizian logic) a different animal. But here I shall venture my own opinion that, if anything stands in the way of this view, it is the violence this concession to the forensic and *C conceptions of persons does to what in real life we actually want to say about amnesiac people.

(4)   The last or commonsensical view is that, *pace* the *C requirement, it is the same person and animal throughout. This is the view that I favor. (176)

Wiggins's criticism of view (1) is correct (although it should be noted that we are rarely, if ever, faced with a case of total amnesia). We would not hold that the concept of person no longer has application in cases of total amnesia. The amnesiac would retain consciousness, beliefs, desires, a subjective perspective on the world, and possibly even a sense of self as a being distinguished from others. Much of the characteristic psychological activity that we associate with the concept of person would still be present. The amnesiac would not be a mere material being.

As argued above, Wiggins is wrong in holding that view (2) is an "incoherent" decision. His own account of the relation between a person and a living human animal as one of constitution and supervenience would allow the same human animal to constitute more than one person over the life history of that animal. Such an appraisal is consistent with the absoluteness of identity, the principle that if a is the same F as b, and a is also a G, then a is the same G as b. Thus, if (2) is to be rejected, it must be for reasons other than that it would violate the absoluteness of identity.

Decision (2) should be rejected because many of the emotional, social, and even legal relationships that existed before the amnesia would persist. The person would retain her property. Love and compassion for the person from relatives and friends would continue, and the person could participate, even at the level of a conscious but passive recipient, in those relationships. In contrast to individuals who have irreversibly lost their subjectivity, such as individuals in PermVS and those who have lost all brain function but may be artificially sustained, the amnesiac retains an ability to enter into conscious, reciprocal relationships with others. This ability may not be sufficient for being a person, but it is minimally necessary.

In addition, many of the biological structures that constituted psychological activity before the amnesia would remain intact through the amnesia. As I argue below, a subjective perspective on the world is tied to physical bodies. The same physical body has persisted through the amnesia, so there is reason to think the same subjective perspective on the world has persisted. If the neurophysiological structures that constitute consciousness and other psychological functions at an earlier time remain intact, what reason would there be for thinking that the consciousness constituted by those same structures belonged to a *different* person at a later time?

The choice between views (3) and (4) reveals fundamental differences in approach to the problem of personal identity. Wiggins correctly construes the choice between (3) and (4) as a choice between functionalist and naturalistic conceptions of persons.

In opposition to decision (3) Wiggins states:

> I think it would be fair to subject an upholder of decision (3) to the following line of questioning: Since you allow the systemic component of the notion of person to dominate the *animal* element completely, and are more sanguine than the last section was intended to encourage anyone to be about the prospects of giving a coherent complete formulation of the psychological or systemic marks of the concept *person*, and since you are anxious to permit a *C condition to invade and reshape the biological principle of individuation of *homo sapiens*, why stop there? Why restrict this concession you have made to the demands of the forensic conception? What import does it have to insist that a person is an *animal* that meets this or that further condition? Why would

you not allow an artifact to qualify as a person, provided it was programmed to satisfy fully the functional requirement that you have claimed to be the principal part of the definition of *person*? Why do you not retreat to a position where the concept *person* is no longer a hybrid concept like *vegetable*, but simply reduces to a complicated functional attribute that is completely specifiable? Seeing the problem of persons in the way you see it, one finds no rationale for choosing any particular point between decision (4), which is the verdict of the biological view of persons (as it is of the replete or naturalistic view that amplifies or enlarges the biological view), and a purely functional conception of persons that will permit an artifact to qualify. Surely decision (3) marks an inherently unstable position, unless we rectify the rationale for it and reformulate this in terms that (in theory at least) allow room for persons who are *not* organisms . . .

I calculate that there is probably no direct argument that will have any efficacy if a philosopher is prepared to count for nothing the illumination that a naturalistic conception can throw upon the perplexity we are caused by thought-experiments involving such things as the interchange of brains or their parts, and the "carbon copy" replication or duplication of skills and memories. For me, or for anyone who is willing to be party to the doctrine of individuation that the naturalistic conception of persons makes possible, it seems immensely important that, at the limit, such thought-experiments denature the human subject, and create the prospect that, in place of an animal or organism with a clear principle of individuation, we shall find some day that we have an entity whose identity has become a matter not of discovery but of interpretation (or even stipulation). (176–78)

I agree to some extent with Wiggins's assessment, but I think he overstates the case. Persons are biological beings, and our understanding of their biology should inform our understanding of their nature. It would be a mistake to treat persons as simply artifacts whose nature is a matter of mere stipulation. Not anything can be a person. Indeed, as with all natural kinds, the lawlike regularities associated with the concept *human being* place restrictions on the possible development of members within its extension. These same restrictions apply to persons insofar as they are constituted by a natural kind. For example, if our neurophysiology tells us that a certain amount of brain matter is required for consciousness, then, assuming that such potential is necessary for something to be a person, human organisms without the requisite neurophysiological structures would be ruled out of the class of persons.

As argued in chapter 4, however, persons are not identical to human organisms and the concept *person* is not a natural kind concept. Because of their essential psychological, moral, and cultural nature, persons are not reducible to their biological being. Our understanding of them is informed not only by biological theory but by psychological, moral, and cultural theories as well. Since psychological, moral, and cultural considerations take us beyond biology, the nature of persons is *in part* a matter of interpretation within those theories. Wiggins thus sets up a false dichotomy by presenting the issue as a choice: thinking of persons as having a nature that is a matter for discovery or having a nature that is subject to interpretation (or even stipulation). Persons are not beings whose nature we can discover in the same way that we can discover that water is H_2O. Nor are persons simply artificial, functional constructions such that the matter constituting them is irrelevant to their individuation and identification. Wiggins comes closest to getting it right when he refers to the concept of person as a "hybrid concept." By this, I interpret him to mean that the concept *person* is determined partly by the biology of the natural kind that constitutes a person and partly by psychological, moral, and cultural considerations. In this interpretation, the fundamental substantial kind under which we are individuated and identified would be neither person *simpliciter* nor human organism. Rather, it would be the hybrid concept *human-person*. Moreover, such a view would make the identity and individuation a matter of arbitrary stipulation only if one thought that one's psychological, moral, and cultural theories were arbitrary. If these theories can have rational support (and I believe they can), then they can provide rational support for our judgments about persons and personal identity.

The treatment of *human-person* as akin to a natural kind concept is also supported by what I believe is the correct interpretation of "multiple personality" or "dissociative personality disorder." If persons are constituted by human organisms in a lawlike way, then there is reason to reject the interpretation of dissociative personality disorder as more than one substantive person being constituted by a human organism. Indeed, in his seminal work on dissociative personality disorder, Morton Prince ([1906] 1969) appealed to a naturalistic view of persons to support his claim that there was only one true person in the body of his patient, Christine Beauchamp.

Before looking at Prince's view in more detail, it is worth noting why one would interpret dissociative personality disorder as a case in which more than one person is constituted by the same human organism. Although Baker does not consider whether multiple persons could be constituted by the same human body, nothing in her view rules out this possibility. In fact, if, as Baker holds, the presence of a strong first-person perspective is sufficient for the individuation of a person, then her view may require that dissociative personality disorder involves more than one person in a single human body. Consider the following exchange between Morton Prince and his patient, Christine Beauchamp, recounted in Prince's seminal work on the disorder:

"Why are you not 'She'?"

"Because 'She' does not know the same things that I do."

"But you both have the same arms and legs, haven't you?"

"Yes, but arms and legs do not make us the same." (Prince [1906] 1969, 27)

Commenting on Prince's work, Kathleen Wilkes (1981) points out that, from the first-person perspective (i.e., what it is like to be someone from the inside), each personality of Christine Beauchamp considered herself separate from the others and was concerned only with her own existence and threatened extinction. Thus, if the personalities have different first-person perspectives, Baker's view seems to entail their being distinct persons.

Prince, however, rejected this interpretation. In his discussion of whether there is one real person or a multiplicity of them, he asserts that assessing persons from simply a psychological point of view, such as from consideration of the strong first-person perspective, is too limited:

Again, approaching the subject from a purely psychological point of view, it has been held that of the various possible selves which may be formed out of the "mass of consciousness" belonging to any given individual, there is no particular real or normal self; one may be just as real and just as normal as another, excepting so far as one or the other is best adapted to a particular environment. If the environment were changed, another self might be the normal one. But the psychological point of view is too limited. What test have we of adaptation? There is a physiological point of view, and also a biological point of view, from which personality must be considered. A normal self must be able to adjust itself physiologically to its environment, otherwise all sorts of perverted reactions of the body arise (anesthesia, instability, neurasthenic symptoms, etc.), along with pathological stigmata (amnesia, suggestibility, etc.), and it becomes a sick self. Common experience shows that, philosophize as you will, there is an empirical self which may be designated the real normal self. However, I shall put aside this question for the present and assume that there is a normal self, a particular Miss Beauchamp, who is physiologically as well as psychologically best adapted to any environment. This self should be free from mental and physical stigmata (suggestibility, amnesia, aboulia, anesthesia, etc.), which commonly characterize the disintegrated states making up multiple personality. Such a self may be termed the real self, in the sense that it is not an artificial product of special influences, but the one which is the resultant of the harmonious integration of all the processes, both physiological and psychological of the individual. Any other self is a sick self. (Prince [1906] 1969, 233–34)

Prince believed that *person*, in its substantive meaning, is a natural kind term, that there are psychological, biological, and physiological laws governing what it is to be a person, and that these laws determine the extension of the term. Some of Beauchamp's personalities (Sally, BI, and BIV) are ruled out as persons because, despite psychological appearances, they violate some natural laws of personhood. Evidence of violation is that they are all "sick" selves.[4]

There is thus substantial agreement between Prince and Wiggins on treating persons as or as "akin to" a natural kind. Wiggins distinguishes artifacts, such as chairs and cups, from natural kinds, or things akin to natural kinds, such as human-persons, on the grounds that the former are not identified under concepts that are nomologically conditioned. Similarly, Prince distinguishes artificial persons from natural persons on the grounds that the former violate the nomological regularities that underlie the concept of person. Both authors maintain that psychological considerations are insufficient to account for our concept of person and that our nature as biological beings is essential to who we are. Finally, both argue for a one-one, person-body relation based on natural laws of psychology, biology, and physiology.

At this point, I wish to note a further disagreement I have with Baker on the nature of the constitutive relation between persons and human organisms. Baker countenances the possibility that a human-person could come to be constituted by a biological being of another species or by a nonbiological being and continue to exist (Baker 2000, 106, 113, 123, 141). In contrast, I believe the constitutive relation between persons and human organisms rules out these possibilities. In her rejection of animalism, Baker considers various thought experiments involving bodily transfer: Locke's famous case of the prince and cobbler swapping bodies, episodes of *Star Trek*, and Kafka's story in which Gregor Samsa wakes up one morning to find himself in the body of a gigantic insect.[5] Baker then argues, "If sameness of person consisted in sameness of living organism, then all of these stories would be not only fictional, but incoherent; what they portray would be not only false, but necessarily false. In that case, why do the stories and thought experiments seem so plausible — so plausible as to tempt some to dualism? Anyone who takes hundreds of years of thought experiments as attempts to depict what is metaphysically impossible should show how so many have gone so badly wrong" (123).

Baker also considers the possibility of a human body being replaced gradually over time by an artificial one:

> Although a human organism could not become a nonbiological being and continue to exist, a human person (originally constituted by a human organism) could come to be constituted by a nonbiological body and still continue to exist. For it may be possible for a human person to undergo gradual replacement of her human body by bionic parts in a way that did not extinguish her first-person perspective; if so, then she would continue to exist but she would cease to have a human body. And she would continue to exist (and to be a person) as long as her first-person perspective remained intact, whether she continued to be constituted by a human body or not. If she came to be constituted by a nonorganic body, then she would no longer be a *human* person. So, a human person is not essentially a human person. (106)

Further, in discussing how the constitutive relation obtains between various kinds of things, Baker contrasts the constitutive relation between Michelangelo's *David* and the marble of which it is made to the constitutive relation between a person and human organism:

> If *x* constitutes *y* at *t*, nothing about constitution per se either precludes or guarantees that *y* could be constituted by something other than *x* in the future at *t'*. Whether or not *y* could come to be constituted by something different from *x* depends on the primary kind of things that *y* is. For example, the persistence conditions of statues differ from those of rivers. If Piece [i.e., the name for a piece of marble] constitutes Michaelangelo's *David* at *t*, I doubt that *David* could exist at *t'* without being constituted by Piece. But if a certain aggregate of molecules constituted a river at *t*, that very river could exist at *t'* without being constituted by that aggregate of molecules. With respect to identity conditions, I believe that persons are more like rivers than statues. I believe that a human person, constituted by a human organism at *t*, could come to be constituted by a bionic body at *t'*. In that case, the person would still exist, although no longer constituted by a human organism. (145)

I disagree. Persons are more like statues than rivers, and a person constituted by a particular human body at one time could not be constituted by a different body, animal or bionic, at a later time. Our human nature is essential (necessary) to the persons that we are. This view, it should be noted, does not entail our being identical to our bodies. Nor does it entail bodily continuity being sufficient for personal identity. It makes *person* neither a natural kind concept nor simply a functional or artifactual concept. Instead, it maintains that bodily continuity is as necessary as our subjectivity in terms of our persistence as the same person over time.

In his discussion of Lot's wife being turned into a pillar of salt, Wiggins (1980, 60–61, 66–67) has challenged the conceivability of such stories on the grounds that the stories, as told, violate laws of nature. If, as suggested above, the fundamental substance concept by which we individuate and identify persons is a hybrid concept (e.g., *human-person*), then the laws governing the extension of the natural kind *human being* restrict the possible development of members within the extension of the hybrid concept. Human-persons are not the kind of thing that can turn into pillars of salt, insects, and so forth. Nor are they the kind of thing that can turn into a robot.

Hans Jonas (1974) also challenges the view that our bodies are not essential to who we are. He questioned what he thought was an underlying brain-body dualism in the move to a brain-based criterion of death. In this form of dualism, which he thought was a revenant of the old, soul-body dualism, "the true human person rests in (or is represented by) the brain, of which the rest of the body is a mere subservient tool" (139). Jonas believes such a view is mistaken:

> Now nobody will deny that the cerebral aspect is decisive for the human quality of life of the organism that is man's . . . But it is no less an exaggeration of the cerebral aspect as it was of the conscious soul, to deny the extracerebral body its essential share in the identity of the person. The body is as uniquely the body of this brain and no other, as the brain is uniquely the brain of this body and no other. What is under the brain's central control, the bodily total, is as individual, and as much "myself," as singular to my identity (fingerprints), as noninterchangeable, as the controlling (and reciprocally controlled) brain itself. My identity is the whole organism, even if the higher functions of personhood are seated in the brain. How else could a man love a woman and not merely her brains? How else could we lose ourselves in the aspect of a face? Be touched by the delicacy of a frame? It's this person's and no one else's. (139)

Finally, Bernard Williams, in his discussion of thought experiments, such as Locke's prince and cobbler swapping bodies, points out some limitations, especially with regard to character and mannerisms, in our ability to imagine such stories (Williams [1970] 1973, 46–47). For example, he wonders how successfully the bodies could express the character of the other person if the persons before the "body swap" were extremely unlike one another psychologically and physically, perhaps even of a different sex. Because the expression of some personal traits or dispositions may be essentially connected with our particular bodies, how could they survive the "swap"? Insofar as they could not, there is some reason for questioning the intelligibility of the story as a bodily exchange of persons. Williams's point is that certain personal traits may be realized only in certain bodies, and this suggests some limitations on the conceivability of the thought experiments. Williams goes on to argue powerfully that we have conflicting intuitions about the thought experiments. Some seem to support thinking of bodily continuity as a criterion for personal identity, whereas others support a psychological continuity criterion. Ultimately, he thinks (and I concur) that the thought experiments are inconclusive.

THE FIRST-PERSON PERSPECTIVE

Another reason for rejecting the possibility of a human being constituting more than one person over its life history appeals to an understanding of persons as subjective beings, beings with a first-person, subjective perspective on the world. In the case of total amnesia or brain zap with recovery of consciousness, the same first-person perspective on the world has not been destroyed, but it is destroyed in cases of PermVS. Some philosophers have argued that this first-person perspective is entirely subjective and unanalyzable from or nonreducible to any objective, third-person point of view (McTaggart 1927, vol. 2, ch. 36; Nagel 1965, 1986; Castañeda 1966; Shoemaker 1968; Block and Fodor 1972; Block 1978, 1980; Madell 1981; Evans 1982, chs. 2 and 7; Jackson 1982; Conee 1985). The first-person perspective can be understood, however, at least in part, as connected to or dependent on the spatiotemporal locations of persons, which can be tracked through time by bodily continuity. Thus, a first-person perspective on the world is a view from somewhere — that is, it is a view from the perspective of wherever the body from which that view emanates happens to be. This perspective does not become a new perspective if a person's bodily location changes or other mental states change. Since the subjective perspective from the body after brain zap is the same perspective as that before brain zap, there is reason for thinking that the same person has persisted through the brain zap.

Baker believes that having a first-person perspective is sufficient for something to be a person at any particular time but that it is impossible to give informative criteria (i.e., sufficient conditions) for personal identity over time without presupposing personal identity. Because the first-person perspective is itself unanalyzable but essential to personal identity, she claims that any reductive account of personal identity in terms of third-person objective criteria is bound to fail (Baker 2000, 118–46). Geoffrey Madell (1981) has argued along similar lines.

I agree with Baker and Madell that subjectivity or the first-person perspective is primitive and irreducible and that having subjectivity or a point of view is necessary for anything to be a person. This precludes the possibility of stating objective, sufficient conditions for personal identity over time. I do not think, however, that this view precludes the possibility of determining some objective, necessary conditions of personal identity. Here I focus on Madell's arguments, which are more explicit than Baker's.

Madell draws on McTaggart's treatment (1927) of *I* as a logically proper name: "The essence of McTaggart's argument is this: If the self can be known only by description, then it cannot be known at all, for unless we were directly aware of ourselves, unless we knew ourselves by acquaintance, we could never tell that any such description applied to us. Even if we allow that two such descriptions could be known to describe one and the same person, it would still be unknown who that person is. I can only know myself to be that one and the same person to whom these various descriptions apply if I have knowledge of myself, an awareness of myself, which is independent of these descriptions" (Madell 1981, 23–24).

As Madell points out, Thomas Nagel (1965, 1986) has reinvoked McTaggart's argument in his claim that there is an area of subjectivity that lies beyond description in physicalist terms. According to Madell, McTaggart and Nagel are pointing to "the gap between descriptions and names on the one hand and first-person ascriptions on the other. No matter how complete the description of what is in fact my body and situation is, there is always a gap between this description and the assertion that it is myself which is thus described. No statement to the effect that there exists a person of such-and-such description could entail that I am that person, nor could it imply it" (Madell 1981, 24). He concludes,

> It seems, therefore, to follow that the proposition that there exists a person satisfying such and such a description, and the proposition that the person thus described is myself, is a purely contingent one, and one which cannot be regarded as evidential either.
>
> McTaggart explicitly draws from these conclusions the conclusion that the property of being a self cannot be analyzed; it is a simple and unanalyzable property like redness. To put it another way, since no description of any body or experience can entail, or otherwise support the claim, that it is mine, the property of being mine is unanalyzable.
>
> It seems to be but a short step from this position to the conclusion that the self as such has no essential properties, apart from "thinking." It happens to be associated with a set of properties, but since nothing about these properties can entail or imply that they are mine it is possible that a quite different set could have been mine, and this is clearly equivalent to saying that the very same self might have been connected with a different set of properties. "I" thus appears to be the name of an unanalyzable entity, an entity with no essential properties except that of thinking or consciousness, an entity whose nature we can grasp in our experience, but which we cannot hope to analyze. (25)

One may agree with McTaggart and Nagel that there is an area of subjectivity that defies physicalist description and that, therefore, the "I" and the connection between the "I" and any description is, at least in part, unanalyzable. Any third-person, empiricist criterion of personal identity is thus insufficient to account for personal identity. It is not "but a short step," however, from the view that no description could entail that description applying to myself to Madell's conclusion that the self has no essential properties. If an essential property is understood in the traditional Aristotelian sense of a property, such that an entity would cease to exist as the kind of thing it is if it lost that property, Madell's inference is mistaken. From the fact that no sufficient conditions can be given for why some property or set of properties are mine, it does not follow that no necessary conditions can be given. Moreover, even if the relation between a person satisfying some description and that person being me is contingent, it does not follow that the relation lacks necessity. The necessity involved may be one of *de re*, empirical necessity or lawfulness.[6]

For example, Madell states that "thinking" or "self-consciousness" may be the only essential property of the "I." Thinking and self-consciousness, however, may have empirically discoverable, essential properties. Thought and self-consciousness may be supervenient events or properties, known by acquaintance, and not identical to any physical events or properties. Nonetheless, their existence may be lawfully dependent on some physical events or properties. In fact, Madell claims that the irreducible, subjective awareness of oneself is, in part, an awareness of oneself as occupying a position in space (Madell 1981, 28). If being an occupant of space is an essential property of the "I," then one would have reason for thinking that the "I" was completely unanalyzable only if one thought that the concept *occupant of space* was also completely unanalyzable. In fact, if physical entities are the only kinds of entities that can occupy space, then being a physical entity would be an essential property of the "I," and knowledge of this essential property would be arrived at partly through one's first-person awareness of one's self. The self or subjectivity would necessarily be identified with a view from somewhere. Moreover, even though the irreducibility of subjectivity would preclude discovery of sufficient, objective criteria for the identity of the self, necessary conditions for the identity and persistence of physical entities might apply to the self.

There is a deeper problem for Madell's view. From the epistemological claim that our first-person knowledge of ourselves at any instant in time is subjective and immune from error through misidentification, the metaphysical claim that the self (or the "I") has no objective conditions for its existence does not follow. I might not need an objective criterion to identify myself, since I have direct, subjective knowledge of who I am at any point in time. This does not imply that what I know subjectively (i.e., the "I") does not have objective conditions of existence, conditions that I may be unaware of in my subjective knowledge of the "I" but which I might later discover.

Madell's failure to distinguish the epistemological claim about how we know the self from the metaphysical claim about the conditions for the existence of the self is apparent in his arguments against the idea that the body is what unites any set of simultaneous experiences in one mind and that bodily continuity is a necessary condition of personal identity.

Madell tries to extend his arguments for the irreducibility and complete unanalyzability of the "I" to show that it is impossible to analyze and state objective criteria for personal identity over time. His initial target is the suggestion that bodily continuity is the criterion of personal identity—that is, the claim that "two or more experiences are the same person's just in virtue of being related to the same body" (Madell 1981, 49). Madell admits that his earlier arguments showed that no analysis is possible of what it is for a group of simultaneous experiences to be the experiences of the same subject, but that it does not obviously follow that no analysis is possible of what it is for experiences through time to be the experiences of the same subject. Jonathan Bennett, for example, believes that although "nothing useful has ever been said about rules or criteria governing the unity of mental states within a single mind-stage," since there can be no problem about what mental states are one's own at any conscious moment, one can have a genuine problem about whether some mental state was one's own (Bennett 1966, 121–22). Bennett thinks the lack of criteria for simultaneous present experiences being one's own does not imply that there can be no criteria for past experiences being one's own.

Madell claims, "It is just not possible to recognize the total absurdity of the suggestion that what unites my present experiences is their being tied to one and the same body, and to continue to hold that what unites my experiences over time is that they are tied to one and the same body" (Madell 1981, 64). Consider two of the arguments he offers in support of his claim. First, he writes, "once it is clear that we have a notion of unity of consciousness which does not depend on the body, a conception that we can get by thinking about the unity which characterizes our present experiences as set, it must also be clear that such unity cannot be confined to the present moment, nor to any single moment. Such unity obtains just as much in the acts of listening to a sentence or tune, experiences which are necessarily spread over time, as it does among simultaneous experiences. Such experiences are not mere conjunctions of events, any more than one's own simultaneous experiences are mere agglomerations of events" (64–65). Second, Madell denies what Bennett and others, including myself, consider a real possibility—that someone can misidentify himself, in the sense that he could claim to have a full and accurate memory of a past incident but be mistaken in supposing that he had the experience in question:

> Now we saw in the case of present experiences such misidentification clearly has to be ruled out; it is not an intelligible possibility. But it may be thought that the case of the past is different: surely I can misremember, and thus misidentify the subject of an experience in the past, in a way in which it is not possible for me to misidentify myself as the subject of a present experience? This, however, is to miss the point. I can have a full and accurate memory of the past action of someone else, but simply misidentify him. This mistake is not due to any inaccuracy in my memory, but to a misinterpretation of the information which came to me at the time and which is retained in my memory. Now the point is that I cannot similarly have a full and accurate memory of an experience of mine, and as a result of some misinterpretation wrongly ascribe that experience to someone else. (66)[7]

There are problems with both of these arguments. First, if, as Madell admits, the "I" is subjectively aware of itself as occupying a position in space, then the unity of conscious experience spread over time, such as listening to a sentence or tune, is partly explained by that experience taking place from a single position or perspective in space. It is inconceivable that the "I" could have two spatiotemporally distinct perspectives on the world when it listens to a sentence or tune. Again, since physical bodies are the kinds of things that occupy space, the unity of experience spread over time is explained, at least in part, by the persistence of a single body and physical perspective on the world. Extending Madell's own claim about what our first-person awareness of ourselves consists of at any particular moment, we can say that our first-person awareness of ourselves over short time frames, such as listening to a sentence or tune, consists in part of an awareness of ourselves as occupying a single spatiotemporally continuous position.

Second, we can and do misidentify ourselves over time. One can claim to remember events that one did not actually witness or experience and that were in fact witnessed or experienced by someone else. One can also dissociate oneself from one's experience over time and attribute to someone else what was one's own experience. In both cases, we resort to a bodily continuity criterion to verify the memory claims. We are not immune from error through misidentification of ourselves in memory, although we cannot be mistaken in our claim that some present experience is ours.

Third, it is unclear why Madell thinks the unanalyzable, subjective awareness of oneself that is immune from error at any particular moment is necessarily preserved in memory. Madell himself separates this unanalyzable self-awareness from memory in his criticism of Parfit's psychological continuity criterion of personal survival. I fear a future pain, according to Madell, not because the person who will experience the pain will have a certain set of memories (the memories I currently have) but because it will be me (unanalyzable me) that will experience the pain. Madell thus believes personal identity is independent of memory, so one presumably would retain the first-person awareness of oneself regardless of what one claimed to remember about oneself. One fears a future pain regardless of whether one correctly identifies oneself in memory. In sum, if the "I" is completely unanalyzable—if nothing can be said about it, and it is just something a person experiences—how Madell can connect it with memory and, in particular, claim that it would be preserved in memory is unclear.

Consideration of what the amnesiac knows when she identifies herself (i.e., when she says, "I don't know who I am") further supports this criticism of Madell's argument. The amnesiac correctly uses the word *I* to refer to herself. Her knowledge of her identity consists of an awareness of a perspective on the world that is her own; she identifies herself from the first-person, subjective point of view. The amnesiac's subjective sense of her identity is the same sense of identity that Madell, McTaggart, Nagel, Baker, and others have claimed is ultimately unanalyzable and cannot be described in objective terms. Again, it provides a person with knowledge of her identity at any given conscious moment but not of her identity over time. Superimposed or built upon this fundamental, subjective knowledge of one's identity is a subjective awareness or knowledge of one's identity over time, what might be called knowledge of one's psychological continuity from a first-person point of view.

The question can now be raised as to what this subjective knowledge of personal identity over time consists of and how it is arrived at. In other words, how does an individual develop a subjective sense of identity over time? How do memories, dispositions, and personality get related to the fundamental subjective awareness of the self to constitute "psychological continuity" and a sense of one's persisting self?

Two different psychological processes seem to be going on. The momentary awareness of oneself is unanalyzable, except that we can say that it consists in part of an awareness of one's existence in space and time and of a particular perspective on the world. Sartre ([1942] 1994, [1945] 1955), Erikson (1956), and Harré (1984), however, tell us that a person's subjective identity over time is dependent on self-conceptions that are in turn dependent on social factors of recognition and reinforcement. Think of games of "peekaboo—I see *you*" that adults play with infants. The child's awareness of herself as herself is dependent on others' awareness of her as a "you." The answers to the questions raised at the end of the preceding paragraph are also questions that are not answered independent of one's relation to others, for our identity is partly determined by how we are regarded by others. Our identity is not individually subjective but depends partly on the subjectivity of the group. For example, the character traits that an individual subjectively identifies as his own may be dependent on others' recognition of their being his. A person may not correctly identify himself with certain traits unless this identification is reinforced or recognized by others. Knowledge of one's identity as a person with certain memories, dispositions, and personality is thus not derived solely from the first-person, subjective experience of oneself that is immune from error through misidentification. I shall have more to say about this social factor below.

In sum, McTaggart, Nagel, Madell, and Baker are correct that there is something irreducible about the self, namely its subjectivity, and that this irreducible subjectivity rules out the possibility of there being any sufficient, empirical, third-person account of the nature of the "I" and personal identity over time. Objective accounts of personal identity or survival, such as a bodily continuity theory and Locke's psychological continuity theory, thus fail to give a complete explanation of what it means for a person to exist at any moment and to persist through time; they fail to account for a person's subjectivity. Madell is mistaken, however, in his claim that the irreducible nature of the self precludes the possibility of stating objective, necessary conditions for the existence and persistence of the self. His own account of subjectivity, as essentially involving an awareness of oneself occupying a position in space, implies that at least one objective, necessary condition of the self can be given—namely, having a physical body and perspective in space. In addition, judgments of one's own identity expressed in memory claims or self-ascriptions of psychological and character traits are not immune from error. Sometimes we need to rely on a third-person perspective, bodily continuity or social recognition, to verify these judgments.

MORAL AND CULTURAL DIMENSIONS OF PERSONS

The "brain zap" case and many other hypothetical cases concerning personal identity have been widely discussed in the philosophical literature. Indeed, the philosophical literature on personal identity over the past fifty years has been dominated by consideration of such puzzling cases. Some, like Eric Olson, have used these "thought experiments" to argue in favor of a bodily continuity theory of personal identity. Derek Parfit has used them to argue for a psychological continuity theory of personal identity but then to suggest that personal survival, rather than personal identity, is all that really matters to us. What is common to these theorists is the assumption that consideration of such hypothetical cases can reveal our intuitions and best judgments about personhood and personal identity. Common to these views is also the assumption that personal identity consists of some internal relation among certain mental or physical states. Thus, for those sympathetic to Locke's view, personal identity consists of psychological continuity among mental states. For those who accept a bodily or brain continuity theory of personal identity, personal identity consists of body or brain continuity. What is most interesting about the brain zap case and many of the other thought experiments, however, as I argue here and in my discussion of Derek Parfit's view in chapter 7, is that they force us to challenge a key assumption in the account of personal identity, accepted by all of these theorists: that personal identity is determined by some internal connection among mental and/or physical states. If persons and personal identity are partly determined by factors external to whatever internal connection may exist among these states—that is, if persons have nonintrinsic properties essentially—then we may gain some insight into how our definition of death is partly determined by factors external to the person who dies. In the case of brain zap, there would be strong pressure from our moral, social, and legal systems of belief to treat the person who suffers brain zap as still alive and as the same person. For example, we would not distribute the person's property according to a last will and testament that the person executed before the brain zap.[8] Similarly, there is strong normative pressure from our moral and legal systems of belief to treat someone with dissociative personality disorder as a single, substantive person (Wilkes 1981).[9] In contrast, if a person has irreversibly lost the capacity or potential for consciousness, these same factors do not support treating the person as still alive.

While I agree with much of what Baker says about how persons are constituted by bodies, my own view of the constitutive relation between persons and human organisms differs in the role that the moral and cultural dimension of persons can play in fixing the boundaries of the concept. Baker takes the presence of what she calls a "strong first-person perspective" as definitive or sufficient for being a person (Baker 2000, 91). She distinguishes between weak and strong grades of first-person phenomena:

> Weak first-person phenomena are exhibited by problem-solving beings whose behavior is explained by attitudes understood perspectivally, from their own points of view. If a dog that exhibits weak first-person phenomena could express its attitudes in English, it would locate things relative to its own spatiotemporal position (e.g., "There is danger over there"). But it would not thereby show that it had any concept of itself or even any ability to recognize itself from a first-person point of view. It simply acts from its own perspective, with itself at the center. All experience of any sentient being is perspectival, had from its own point of view. It is characteristic of weak first-person

phenomena that they are perspectival in this way. The dog has conscious states like pain and dispositional states like beliefs and desires about its present environment, but it cannot conceive of itself in the first-person as the subject of those states.

On the other hand, strong first-person phenomena require that the subject conceptualize the distinction between himself (and everything else) from a third-person point of view and himself from a first-person point of view. The subject of strong first-person phenomena is not only able to attribute to himself first-person thoughts (typically, using "I"), but is also able to attribute to himself first-person thoughts (typically, using "I*"). Not only can he think of himself, but he can also think of himself*. He can consciously entertain thoughts and conceive of his thoughts as his own*. (67)

According to Baker, an important feature of the strong first-person perspective is that it is relational: "it would be impossible for a being truly alone in the universe to have a first-person perspective" (69–70). She elaborates: "One cannot think of oneself as oneself* without concepts of other things by means of which to distinguish things as being different from oneself; and one cannot have concepts of other things without the presence of other things. It is only over and against other things in the world that one stands as subject with a first-person perspective" (72). At this point, Baker states, she agrees with P. F. Strawson's claim in *Individuals* (1959) that "a condition of the ascription of states of consciousness to oneself is ability to ascribe them to others" (Baker 2000, 72). This feature of the first-person perspective supports Baker's claim that persons, like works of art, have nonintrinsic essential properties. If persons can exist only in relation to others (i.e., in a social context), then their identity and individuation are, in part at least, determined by others.

I agree with Baker's account of the difference between strong and weak first-person phenomena and her claim that persons are partly constituted by relational properties, but I disagree that having a strong first-person perspective is sufficient for being a person. Consider, for example, the amnesiac who wakes up, looks in the mirror, and says, "I don't know who I am." In such an expression, the individual exhibits strong first-person phenomena. The second use of *I* in the sentence requires the ability to conceive of oneself as distinct from other things in the world and as the bearer of intentional states. It is unclear, however, that this would be sufficient for personhood. Suppose this were all that the amnesiac could do. Suppose the amnesiac went on living with such momentary strong first-person awareness of himself but had lost all ability for short- and long-term memory and also the ability to relate different intentional states of himself and others to the same "I" over time. While this individual would have momentary awareness of himself as distinct from others, his knowledge of himself would lack content. Such an individual would clearly lack much of the self-reflective abilities that most of us enjoy, abilities that are critical for our having concern about our past and future and acting as a moral agent. Indeed, as Rom Harré (1984) suggests, some forms of senility may involve this type of restricted strong first-person phenomena.

It is also unclear how others would relate to an individual with such a limited sense of self. If the individual is incapable of recollecting and projecting his self, in what sense can the individual be said to have a personal life, an autobiography? Indeed, if such an individual is viewed as having a personal life, it will not be solely by virtue of his having a strong first-person perspective. It will be because others provide a social and cultural context for recognition of the individual as a person. Others are able to fill in the autobiographical history and may continue to treat the individual as the same person, for various reasons. They may continue to care for him, partly because of the emotional ties that continue to bind. The individual can continue to experience the world and have desires and interests, and others may recognize those interests and desires and sympathize with their satisfaction. Even though the capacity for moral agency may be lost, since the individual cannot remember the past and project into the future, enough of the psychological systemic component essential to the person remains. Elements of weak first-person perspective also persist, so the individual cannot be treated as a mere material being, a thing.

The underlying problem with taking the strong first-person perspective as sufficient for personhood is that it ignores the essential nature of persons as social beings. Having a strong first-person awareness of ourselves is not enough. As Harré points out, "If experiencing matters as one's own were only an ephemeral or momentary phenomenon, then this would not yield the full sense of personal uniqueness. There has also to be some kind of experiential continuity. In some ways or other, an individual woman, for example, must treat most of her actions as developments of and connected with her past personal experience and as attributes of one being, herself. In short, a person's present actions must be located in an autobiography, representing the past and anticipating the future" (Harré 1984, 204).

Developing P. F. Strawson's insight on how our sense of personal identity is tied to bodily considerations and our recognition (or interpretation) of other persons, Harré suggests our social being is reflected in our system of personal pronouns and how we come to use them:

> The indexicality of "I" depends, it might be argued, upon the grasp of the simple referential function of "you." Since "myself" is not a thing I could discover, it seems I cannot first experience myself and then attach the personal pronoun "I" to that experience. I must be learning the pronoun system as a whole through the ways in which and the

means by which I am being treated as a person by others. So that, by being treated as "you," or as a member of "we," I am now in a position to add "I" to my vocabulary, to show where, in the array of persons, speaking, thinking, feeling, promising and so on, is happening. In order to be addressed as "you," I must be being perceived as a definite embodied person, that is, as a distinct human but material individual by others. This unity of the pronoun system might be one of the things that is meant by the social construction of the self. But it depends upon the recognizable bodily identity that I have even as an infant. I have identified these as the indexical uses of "I." (Harré 1984, 211)

Harré further observes that we are treated by other people as having a distinct point of view and as being a locus of agency. The very conditions of bodily identity that are necessary conditions for having the idea of ourselves as persons are, he states, "embedded in all kind of social practices . . . in such practices as moral praise and blame" (211). He concludes,

So the acquisition of the idea of a personal identity for oneself, through which one develops a sense of identity, is at least in part a consequence of social practices which derive from the fact of identity as it is conceived in a culture. Our first preliminary conclusion, then, must be that a human being learns that he or she is a person from others and in discovering a sphere of action the source of which is treated by others as the very person they identify as having spatiotemporal identity. Thus, a human being does not learn that he or she is a person by the empirical disclosure of an experiential fact. Personal identity is symbolic of social practices not of empirical experiences. It has the status of a theory. (212)

Harré's point that personal identity is, at least in part, a matter of social and cultural interpretation and practice and not purely an empirical fact to be discovered is significant to the problem of defining and determining death. If social and cultural factors inform our sense of personal identity, then those same factors are relevant when we are confronted with cases that challenge whether some individual should be counted among the living "we." The point of considering the possibility of someone having a severely limited, yet momentary, strong first-person perspective is not to suggest that such an individual would necessarily fall outside the bounds of personhood. Rather, if we were to continue to treat this individual as a person, we would not do so simply because of the presence of a strong first-person perspective. It would be because we can sympathize with the individual and are willing to extend compassion and recognition.

The situation is much different when we consider an individual in PermVS or one who has lost all brain function. *If* these individuals have lost their ability to experience the world, they have lost their subjectivity and hence fall outside the boundaries of persons. They are mere material beings. Sympathy, compassion, and social recognition are no longer appropriate responses. This, of course, does not mean that these individuals should not be treated with some respect, but the respect accorded to them should be more in line with the respect we accord to corpses. Sympathy and compassion are inappropriate moral responses to corpses. Corpses lack feeling and interests, so there is nothing to sympathize with. The same can be said about our relation to individuals in PermVS and those who have lost all brain function.

We should note that the inappropriateness of sympathy, compassion, and other moral emotions in these cases is predicated on the belief that these human organisms have lost their potential and capacity for subjectivity. This belief, of course, is based on an assumption that subjectivity in human organisms is dependent on certain brain functions and that those functions are irreversibly destroyed in cases of PermVS and whole-brain-dead human organisms. If one were to reject these assumptions, then the responses of sympathy and compassion toward these individuals and other moral beliefs about them might be appropriate. For example, as discussed in the next chapter, D. Alan Shewmon rejects the assumption that the potential for consciousness and other mental functions resides in the brain. According to Shewmon, individuals who have lost all brain function still retain the potential for intellect and will and, therefore, they have not died. This view is based on a specific understanding of potentiality—one that I believe we have good reason to reject but that Shewmon believes is supported by the Catholic philosophical and theological tradition.

Other examples of how different metaphysical beliefs embedded in cultural practices may affect whether an individual is treated as a living person are reflected in why some Japanese, Jewish, and American Indian peoples reject whole-brain death as death. Some members of these groups believe the spirit has not left the body as long as respiration is present, regardless of whether respiration is maintained by natural or artificial means. They understand death as the separation of the spirit from the body, and death has not occurred until respiration has ceased. For example, the traditional Japanese concept of *kokoro* as an "inner" stable self or core of the person may play a role in why some Japanese people reject brain death as death. Lock (2002, 227–28) explains that *kokoro* is thought to lie in the depths of the body, but it is not an anatomical organ. It is neither identified with the brain nor associated exclusively with the mind. Yet it is regarded as the source of the stable "inner" self or person. Since *kokoro* may be thought to remain even in a body that has lost all brain function, some Japanese do not accept brain death as death. Finally, Vera Kalitzkus points out that in Hinduism, *atman*, or the soul, is not released from the body until the main mourner, usually the eldest son, smashes the skull of the person who has undergone cremation: "With the postponement of the final point of death to the smashing of the skull, death falls under the control of the social: it is transferred from the realm of the natural to that of the cultural" (Kalitzkus 2004, 144).

The point of these examples is to show how different metaphysical beliefs are embedded in different cultural practices and how those practices affect whether and when a person is treated as dead. People will continue to differ on whether and when certain individuals should be considered dead, because they will continue to differ on their view of the nature of persons. I am not suggesting that we should accept a naive relativism about persons or that cultural practice cannot be changed. The new types of cases created by advances in medical technology should force us to reflect on our beliefs and practices and, for some cases, to revise them. Thus, on reflection, we may determine that some practices are inconsistent with other things we believe about persons and how they should be treated. The practices may also be based on mistaken beliefs about other matters. For example, in the next chapter I try to show that Shewmon and others rely on a mistaken view about potentiality in their arguments for rejecting neurological criteria for determining death. Indeed, a view that treats persons as constituted by material beings (in our case, human organisms) and as essentially having a subjective, moral, and social nature is inconsistent with treating as persons those human organisms that have irreversibly lost the capacity for subjectivity.

At this point, it should be clear what is wrong with Veatch's criticism of Green and Wikler's view (see chapter 3). Veatch's error lies in his assumption that, in all or most theories of personhood and personal identity, individuals with severe dementia or complete amnesia have lost their personhood or personal identity. Again, we need to be careful in identifying whether we are referring to theories invoking the "qualitative meaning" or "substantive meaning" of person. While Veatch may be correct that some theories of the person, in both senses of the term, link personhood to some relatively high level of autonomous, rational activity and thus would be committed to the view that the person with dementia has ceased to exist, this is not true of all theories. Since individuals with dementia may retain many of the psychological functions that we ordinarily associate with persons—for example, they perceive, feel, have some memories and awareness of themselves over time, have some interests, and may have limited concern for their immediate future—some theories of personhood might not rule out these individuals from the class of persons. In P. F. Strawson's view, for example, psychological predicates would still be attributable to these individuals, and thus they would not be mere material beings. Similarly, Wiggins's neo-Lockean activity-grounded principle for the individuation of persons would be satisfied to a certain degree, and thus, again, individuals with dementia would not necessarily be ruled out of the class of persons. More to the point, since Veatch argues for a consciousness-related formulation of death, on the grounds that it coheres best with his Judeo-Christian tradition, it is unclear why he assumes the qualitative view of personhood, rather than the substantive view that I believe is central to that tradition. The hypothetical case of brain zap can thus be accommodated in a theory that (1) understands death as something that literally happens to persons and (2) avoids the unacceptable implication that a death has occurred with brain zap.

In addition, if persons and personal identity are partly determined by factors external to the body of the person, then it is legitimate to appeal to such factors to resolve problematic cases. In the case of brain zap, there would be strong pressure from our moral, social, and legal systems of belief to treat the person as still alive and as the same person. For example, as noted earlier, we would not distribute the person's property according to a last will and testament that the person executed before the brain zap. Moreover, the same person persists through the hypothetical case of brain zap because consciousness and a particular first-person perspective on the world have not been destroyed. This perspective does not become a new perspective if a person's bodily location changes or if her other mental states change. Thus, since the subjective perspective from the body after brain zap is the same as that before brain zap, we have reason to think that the same person has persisted through the brain zap.

CHAPTER SIX

Persons as Human Organisms

Critics of a consciousness-related formulation of death who employ the "species meaning" of person, such as Capron, Olson, and Feldman, can (unlike Bernat, Culver, and Gert) consistently maintain that the person continues to exist in cases of permanent vegetative state (PermVS). Since these theorists identify the person with the human organism, they claim that, when we point to the individual in PermVS, we are referring to the "person" and not simply the "human being." Also, in this view (and again, unlike that of Bernat, Culver, and Gert), *death* can be predicated literally to persons. For example, since Alexander Capron identifies the person with the biological organism and believes death is primarily a biological concept, persons are the kind of thing that can literally die.

These "species meaning" theorists, however, make the same kind of mistake as Bernat, Culver, and Gert: in their dismissal of the consciousness-related, neurological formulation of death, they employ a concept of person that would be rejected by proponents of the personhood argument who favor that formulation. As noted in chapter 3, Capron (1987) holds that "the accepted criterion for being considered a person is live birth of the product of a human conception." Philosophers from Boethius to Lynne Rudder Baker, however, have linked personhood to a being with the capacity or, at least, the potential for some psychological functions. Thus, to hold a view about the definition of death that treats as persons those individuals who lack the potential or capacity for consciousness or any other psychological functions departs from the traditional philosophical understanding of *person* in its "substantive meaning" sense.

Moreover, invoking a "species meaning" sense of person to claim that the "personhood argument" in favor of a consciousness-related formulation of death is mistaken and that the person in PermVS has not died is to fail to address the force of the argument. Since proponents of the personhood argument use *person* in its substantive meaning to refer to a human being with the capacity or potential for consciousness, to attack it on the grounds that the person in PermVS still exists in a "species meaning" sense is to attack a straw man. Proponents of the personhood argument could agree that the person in a "species meaning" sense still exists in PermVS. They claim, however, that the person in a "substantive meaning" sense has died.

As Christopher Gill (1990a, 156) points out, David Wiggins has suggested that our concept of person tries to hold together "in a single focus" three different ideas or aspects of *person:*

1. an object of biological, anatomical, and neurophysiological inquiry;
2. a subject of consciousness; and
3. a locus of all sorts of moral attributes and the source or conceptual origin of all value.[1]

Wiggins's approach is helpful because it suggests that, when faced with problematic cases that challenge the range of our concept of person, such as the whole-brain dead, individuals in PermVS, or human embryos, we need to examine to what extent these beings are like ourselves in the three senses that inform our concept of person. We also need to examine how these three features are interconnected. Too often, theorists focus on one of these aspects and ignore the others. This is particularly evident in the philosophical discussion about personal identity over the past fifty years. Much paper has been spent debating whether personal identity consists of bodily or psychological continuity, with little consideration about the moral dimension of persons and personal identity. The thought experiments that challenge our concept of persons and personal identity tend to sunder persons from the cultural and moral context in which they appear. If Wiggins is right, we should not expect to have a purely metaphysical or value-free account of the nature of a person.

Commenting on Wiggins's three aspects of persons, Christopher Gill observes that the key to Wiggins's account is "the idea of interpretation":

> These ideas of the person are intelligible to us because, and in so far as, we deploy (or at least presuppose) them in the process of interacting with, and making sense of, other

human beings.[2] Similarly, it is worthwhile for us as thinkers to try to hold these different ideas "in a single focus," because, in our ordinary relationships with other human
beings, we are capable of treating them as "persons" in the three relevant senses, and
of doing so in an interconnected way.

A crucial point in Wiggins's argument is that this type of interpretation is mutual
and reciprocal. Human beings, considered as persons, "are subjects of fine-grained interpretations *by* us and are the would-be exponents of fine-grained interpretations *of*
us." We interpret persons, that is to say, as beings like ourselves (and as capable of interpreting us as beings like themselves); and this fact has implications for our understanding of human beings as persons in all three of the senses Wiggins identifies as well
as in their interconnection. In particular, it helps to explain the moral scruple with
which we treat those we regard as persons: we think of them as being (like ourselves)
consciousness-bearing, embodied individuals, capable of originating action and of in-
teracting with us as persons. This explains our proper sense of moral constraint at the
thought of treating a human being as a thing, or non persons, whose presence can be
ignored or (at worst) deleted by willful killing. (Gill 1990a, 156)

Thus, in evaluating our intuitions about borderline cases and whether we should
treat persons as phases of human organisms, as identical to human organisms (even
dead ones, as some have suggested), or as constituted by human organisms, we need
to bear in mind this interpretive task. We need to ask whether and to what extent
these alternative accounts of personhood do justice to our understanding of ourselves as biological, conscious, and moral beings. As I have argued in chapters 4 and
5, a substantive concept of person that understands persons as constituted by but not
identical to human organisms provides the best theoretical framework for bringing
together these three different ideas of what it is to be a person.

In this chapter, I provide additional support for accepting this substantive view of
persons over the species view. The substantive view agrees with the species view that
persons are biological beings, but the views part company over the sense in which
persons *are* biological beings. In the species view, *is* in sentences such as "A person
is a human being or human organism" gets interpreted as identity, but substantive
theorists may interpret the *is* in the sense of constitution, as outlined in chapter 5.
Support for this constitutive interpretation comes from the idea that persons are essentially subjective beings, but this is not necessarily true of all human organisms.
Although Baker regards a strong first-person perspective as necessary for personhood, weakening this requirement to a weak first-person perspective would still exclude from the class of persons individuals in PermVS and artificially sustained,
whole-brain-dead human organisms. Support for the substantive view also comes

from consideration of persons as moral beings. I focus on these aspects as reasons for rejecting the species view.

ANIMALISM

Little thought seems to have been given to the moral implications of identifying ourselves with human organisms, dead or alive. For example, David Mackie (1999) observes that the formulation of animalism that identifies the person with the human organism in Fred Feldman's "dead or alive" sense invites the question "who are 'we'?" He then states, "To this question, the answer must be that 'we' means you, me, and those persons who are of the same substantial kind as us" (Mackie 1999, 230). Since Mackie and Feldman identify persons with members of the biological kind *Homo sapiens* and they believe human corpses are still members of that biological kind, they count human corpses among the "we."[3] One wonders what company Feldman and Mackie keep! They seem not to have the "discomfort" that Wiggins says most of us feel about any straightforward identification of ourselves with our bodies. They also ignore the relevance of subjectivity and reciprocity that Wiggins, Gill, Harré, and others identify as central to personhood.

There are contexts in which we intelligibly refer to human corpses as "dead persons." The detective investigating a multiple murder might report, "There are three dead people in the third-floor apartment." At a funeral, someone might say, "We're burying Grandma today." At Italian wakes, someone is always turning around and remarking how good Grandma looks. There are also contexts, as noted in chapter 3, when we use the term *person* to refer to human bodies, regardless of whether they are alive or not (e.g., a sign in an elevator reads, "Maximum capacity: six persons"). These linguistic practices, however, simply reflect that the term *person* is not univocal. In addition, we should note how much we do *not* say about corpses or human bodies that we do normally say about living, conscious persons. For example, we do not attribute the normal range of moral predicates to human corpses. Concepts such as autonomy, freedom, and responsibility, or loving, sensitive, and angry, and so forth, are simply inapplicable. We can also substitute other expressions for *person* in some of these contexts without loss of meaning. For example, "We're burying Grandma today" can be more clearly expressed by "We're burying the remains of Grandma today." In contrast, substituting, say, "The remains of the president are addressing the nation this evening" for "The president is addressing the nation this evening" makes no sense.

Wiggins's observation about the discomfort we feel about any straightforward identification of ourselves with our bodies can be extended to the discomfort most people would feel if they were asked whether they would identify themselves with their artificially sustained, decapitated body. Most people would say that such human organisms would not be them, and they would not include such beings among the "we." If we relax the condition to allow for the human head to remain but with no brain function, then again, most people would not identify themselves with such beings and would not count these individuals among the "we." The same could be said of many people's intuitions about anencephalics and individuals in PermVS, although I suspect there may be more uncertainty about these cases. This uncertainty may have to do mostly with an uncertainty about whether individuals in PermVS or anencephalics have any potential for consciousness.

When we turn to human organisms that have the potential for consciousness and other mental functions or who demonstrate minimal awareness and sentience, there is much greater disagreement about whether to include them among the "we."

Consideration of the moral significance of sentience and of potentiality complicates matters. Few moral theories accord *any* moral standing (never mind the moral standing we accord to persons) to beings that utterly lack the potential for consciousness, awareness, and sentience (Warren 2000).[4] Indeed, some theorists, like Shewmon and Seifert, wish to accord moral standing to the artificially sustained, whole-brain dead because they assume that these individuals still have a potential for intellect and will. More theorists would assign some moral value to beings with consciousness and sentience, since sentience usually implies a capacity to experience pleasure and pain and that capacity may imply the existence of a subject with some rudimentary interests. Utilitarian theorists, for example, would consider such beings in their moral calculations. But, even if the potential or capacity for sentience were assigned some moral value, it would still be an open question whether these features would be sufficient for the high moral standing that is usually accorded to persons.

Our initial intuitions about whether we should count individuals in PermVS and the artificially sustained, whole-brain dead as among the "we" may thus receive support from more reflective, moral considerations. While Feldman is right that consideration of the biological structure of dead specimens of the human species may lead us to consider them to be human beings or persons (are not butterflies carefully preserved and mounted still butterflies?), biological structure is only one aspect of human beings and persons. Unless we think our ontology is completely independent of having a perspective on the world, values, and interests, there is no reason why these biological aspects should take precedence over the psychological and moral aspects of persons.

Whether anencephalics, individuals in PermVS, and the artificially sustained, whole-brain dead are persons may thus vary according to one's moral theory. Here, the question of whether they are persons may not be readily answered by some discovery about the nature of persons. Because *person* is not a univocal term and there is no universally agreed upon theory about the nature of persons, it may be possible to criticize alternative views about persons only by showing how those views conflict with the rules of usage of the terms within a given theory of personhood or how they conflict with other accepted ethical or metaphysical beliefs. In other words, the question may be answered by how consistent our application of the term is with other things that we want to say about persons. If our moral theory assumes that organisms worthy of moral concern must minimally be able to experience the world and that such experience is minimally required to gain the moral status that the theory normally accords to persons, then individuals lacking the potential to experience the world would not be persons.

Adherents to various theories of personhood can draw the line of death at the point of irreversible loss of consciousness and all cognitive function. The death of the person would occur in cases of amentia but not dementia. Indeed, while philosophers in the Western tradition have disagreed over which particular psychological characteristics are sufficient for being a person, the tradition evinces a strong commitment to the view that at least some psychological characteristics, or the potential for some, are minimally necessary.[5]

POTENTIALITY AND DEATH

In the recent literature, several Catholic scholars, including Joseph Seifert and D. Alan Shewmon, have rejected any neurological criterion for determining death—including the loss of all brain function—because they seem to reject any distinction between the person and the human organism.[6] Their grounds for rejecting this distinction are confusing. For example, Seifert (1993) seems to reject the distinction primarily on pragmatic grounds: the pragmatic reason of wishing to avoid the error of mistaking a human person for a nonperson. His view is that, in cases such as anencephaly and PermVS, it is indeterminate whether the human organism has the potential for consciousness and other cognitive functions, and therefore we lack the "moral certainty" to conclude that these human organisms are not persons or that they have died.[7] Instead, we should assume that they are persons. Shewmon (1997), by contrast, offers metaphysical considerations for identifying the person with the human organism. He argues that, even if a human organism has irreversibly lost all brain functions, it still retains the potential for intellect and will, and it therefore is still a person. The difference is important. If the identification of the person with the living human organism is pragmatic rather than metaphysical, then the assumption that all human organisms are persons may be defeated in some cases, and no conceptual impossibility would be involved in holding that some human organisms are not persons or that a person may die even though the organism remains alive. I argue that this is the case for Seifert, and I challenge Shewmon's claim that a human organism that retains somatic integration but has irreversibly lost all brain function would still have the potential for intellect and will. Shewmon relies on a problematic concept of potentiality to sustain his claim. A more sensible, realistic concept of potentiality would support the claims that the life histories of persons and human organisms can diverge and that a person can die even though the organism that constituted it may remain alive. These claims do not require acceptance of the secular arguments involving the *is* of constitution but can be supported by what William Wallace (1995) has called Thomas Aquinas's view of "early dehominization."

Seifert stops short of strictly identifying the person with the human organism, even though he seems to reject any separation of the life history of the person from that of the human organism. Thus, after stating that he is following the Platonic tradition of defining death as "the separation of the soul from the body," Seifert writes,

> But is it not obvious that there must be some distinction between biological and personal human life—especially in view of the divisibility and lack of strict individuality of biological life-processes and genetic codes versus the absolute indivisibility of the mind? There is indeed a distinction here. Yet admitting this difference does not force us to admit the separability of man's soul from his vegetative and sensitive life and to assume the possibility of living human vegetables from whom the soul has left. On the contrary, the close union between personal human life and the biological life of the human organism as a whole is obvious. As long as the biological life of man as a whole is present, we have, in virtue of the unity of body and soul in man and in virtue of the profound formation of the human body by the human spirit, *the best reason to assume* the presence of the personal human mind. In fact, death in the biological sense is without any doubt intimately tied up, either as its cause or as its consequence, with the parting of the mind from the body. Since biological human life is so closely united with man's personal life and since it can be more directly observed, it is this which must serve as our criterion in medicine . . .
>
> It is difficult, however, to maintain any form of strict identity of rational soul and the principle of vegetative/biological life, because biological life does not require one identical and indivisible subject. It is found in each organ and cell which can be isolated in cell-cultures, etc. The "live heart" can be preserved after the obvious death of

the patient. Thus, at least on the level of single biological life processes, strict identity of the subject which gives rational and vegetative life to man seems impossible to maintain. In this sense, we recognize a real difference between the human soul and the biological life-processes. (Seifert 1993, 184–87, emphasis added)

Seifert's position is contradictory. If he admits the distinction between biological and personal life, then he must at least countenance the *possibility* "of living human vegetables from whom the soul has left." Indeed, it is unclear why he thinks such a possibility is any less conceivable than the possibility of human corpses from which the soul has left. Rather than denying the possibility of a personal life ending separately from the biological life with which it was "substantially united," Seifert may only be warranted in claiming that, for the practical task of medically declaring death, we should *assume* that the biological and personal human life cannot diverge. Indeed, he goes on to develop this view by arguing that we lack the moral certainty necessary for concluding that the rational soul has departed from a human body when all brain function has been lost.

Seifert would thus be critical of Paul Ramsey's acceptance (1970) of a neurological criterion on the grounds that Ramsey was mistaken, not about the nature of persons but in concluding that the artificially sustained, brain-dead human organism was merely a collection of organic parts. Seifert holds that enough organized life remains that the human organism continues to exist as a whole and we should therefore assume that the person continues to exist as a whole. According to Seifert, while Ramsey was right about the nature of personhood and misinterpreted the clinical facts, others err in accepting a neurological criterion because they have a mistaken view about persons.

Seifert's metaphysical targets are what he calls (1) a neo-Cartesian dualism of entrances and exits of substantial souls in human bodies and (2) a body-mind identity theory or an epiphenomenalism. He states that one or the other of these views usually underlies acceptance of a neurological criterion for death. His rejection of the materialism inherent in (2) is understandable given his theological assumptions. These assumptions also explain why he rejects the species meaning that, say, Feldman accepts. His rejection of view (1) is more problematic. While he seems to reject (1) because it does not do justice to the idea of a substantial union of the mind and body in the human being, he states that he is following Plato in understanding death as the separation of the soul from the body.[8] Acceptance of death as the separation of the soul from the body, however, and rejection of a strict identification of the person (rational soul) with a vegetative/biological life must allow for the possibility that personal and organic life may diverge. In addition, as I discuss further below,

Wallace (1995) has shown how the acceptance of a consciousness-related formulation of death is consistent with Aquinas's hylomorphic conception of the human being.

Shewmon's position on the criteria for determining death has evolved from initially accepting (1985) a neocortical criterion or "higher-brain" formulation of death to his rejection (1997, 1998a, 1998b) of any neurological criterion and insistence on circulatory-respiratory criteria.

In his 1985 article, Shewmon argued on Aristotelian and Thomistic principles that, in the severest cases of persistent vegetative state and dementia, "what remains is no longer the body of a *person*" (48). Invoking Aquinas's view that, for a rational soul to inform a human body, the *organ* of the internal senses (brain) must be able "to support the proper functioning of the spiritual intellect" (Shewmon 1985, 53),[9] he reasoned that "there is no *a priori* reason to exclude the possibility of a higher level soul being superseded by a lower level soul, rather than by a mixture of inanimate forms" (41).[10] He suggested that there could be "substantial transformations from one level of life to another" (43). Persons (i.e., rational souls informing matter) are different kinds of things from animals (animal souls informing matter) and vegetables (vegetative souls informing matter). Consistent with Thomistic principles, one kind of living being, such as a person, could be substantially transformed into another kind of living being, such as what Shewmon called a "humanoid" animal. He thus construed the change resulting from persistent vegetative state and severe dementia as "the death of the person, even though there is still a humanoid animal body left behind" (59).

In Shewmon's 1997 article, he seems to abandon these principles about the nature of persons and substantial change. He now argues that, even if the entire brain has been destroyed, the person may still be alive, "because the potency for these specifically human functions resides—ultimately—in the organism and not the organ" (74). Absent from this later article is any discussion of why he no longer countenances the possibility of one kind of living substance, a person, changing into another kind of living substance, such as a humanoid animal. Instead, he invokes a questionable notion of "potency" in order to rule out this possibility, which he correctly identified in his earlier work. After reviewing his argument, I will explain why his notion of "potency" is so problematic.

Shewmon rhetorically asks, "Is the incapacity to regenerate a new brain truly a loss of the potency for specifically human properties, i.e., a loss of the human essence, or merely an impediment to the actualization of such potency existing on a deeper level?" In response, he claims that it is merely an accidental impediment and that the human essence is not lost. He offers an analogy in support of his view:

"Consider the function of sight. A century ago dense bilateral cataracts would have produced permanent, irreversible blindness. But such irreversibility was not absolute or intrinsic to the blind person; it was extrinsic, conditional upon the state of the art of ophthalmology. From a metaphysical standpoint, the potency to see was not really lost but persisted in the integrity of the retina, optic nerves and brain and nowadays its re-actualization following cataract surgery is routine." Shewmon then extends the example to include enucleation of both eyes and removal or infarction of the entire visual cortex. He still claims that the person would not have lost the potency to see, which he asserts is "rooted in the very being of the living organism" (Shewmon 1997, 73).

Shewmon then applies this same reasoning to the loss of the brain:

> As with potency for sight, the potency for these functions [human intellection and will] ultimately resides not in the organ, but in the organism. Theoretically, if brains could be reconstituted (e.g., through implanted futuristically transformed neuroblasts), a "brain-dead" person could be made to regain consciousness and other human functions, although perhaps with a clean mnemonic slate and new personality traits (depending on the details of the new synaptic network) . . .
>
> If we understand "person" in the traditional, more substantive way (the enduring substrate of changeable personality traits, memories, reasoning power, etc.), then it follows from everything above that as long as the human body is alive (from the biological perspective of somatic integrative unity) then the person is alive, even if the person's mental functions be paralyzed by a brain lesion, because the potency for these specifically human functions resides—ultimately—in the organism and not the organ . . .
>
> Thus, if "brain death" does not cause loss of somatic integrative unity (as it now seems not to), then neither does it cause a loss of essential human properties, i.e., a loss of potency for specifically human functions—potency at the most profound ontological level, at which the occurrence or not of substantial change is determined . . . (74–75)

Shewmon thus holds that being a "living" member of the human biological species is sufficient for being a person, since all such beings, including the whole-brain dead and, say, an artificially sustained, decapitated human body, have the potency for the specifically human functions of intellect and will. At this point, however, he departs from his earlier Aristotelian and Thomistic principles and invokes a notion of potency or potentiality that is conceptually problematic and useless.

Aristotle (*Metaphysics* 9.7.1048b35–1049b1) recognizes degrees of potentiality. In a remote sense, any matter is potentially anything. Joel Feinberg (1974) makes a similar observation when he asks us to consider the potential of a pile of dehydrated orange juice. The powder is potentially orange juice (just add water) but is potentially many other things as well. All we have to do is adjust the conditions. For example, since we could add water and arsenic, it is potentially poison. Since we could add flour, eggs, and yeast, and then bake, it is potentially orange cake. Feinberg correctly observes that this sense of *potentiality* is so "promiscuous" as to be practically useless.

The more reasonable and proximate, Aristotelian sense of potentiality is one in which matter is organized in such a way that, in the natural or normal course of events, certain potentials are likely to be actualized. For example, acorns have the potential to become oak trees, but acorns have the potential to become oak trees in a "fuller" sense only after they are planted. Thus, in answer to the question of whether earth is potentially man, Aristotle answers, "No—but rather when it has already become seed, and perhaps not even then. It is just as it is with being healed; not everything can be healed by the medical art or by luck, but there is a certain kind of thing which is capable of it, and only this is potentially healthy" (Aristotle *Metaphysics* 9.7.1049a1–4).[11] Aristotle's point is that these more proximate or realistic potentials exist only if some "requisite antecedents" obtain in the substance and the world. In the same vein, Aristotle (*Nicomachean Ethics* 2.1.1103a15–1103b25) holds that one has the potential to act virtuously only if one has received the appropriate training—that is, only if some condition extrinsic to the human being has been met and the human being has been modified. All human beings may have the potential to be trained to act virtuously, but it is senseless to attribute this more realistic sense of potential to act virtuously to someone who has not been so trained. This latter potential does not exist unless the antecedent conditions have been met.

Aristotle thus rules out certain potentials because the requisite antecedents are lacking in the substance; for example, acorns do not have the potential to become pine trees, or someone's condition is such that it cannot be healed. In all cases, whether a potential exists depends on whether it can be actualized, where "can be actualized" is dependent not only on the internal state of the substance but also on external conditions. Privation in the internal state of the substance or in external conditions that cannot be rectified in any realistic way is grounds for concluding that the substance lacks certain potentials in this more proximate or realistic sense.

Moreover, Aristotle would distinguish those cases in which it simply *is not* up to us whether a potential can be actualized from those cases in which it *is* up to us. On the one hand, for example, we currently lack the knowledge and technology to alter the genes of an acorn so that it could develop into a pine tree, so acorns do not have any realistic potential to develop into pine trees. Similarly, we lack the knowledge and technology to heal certain conditions, so patients in those conditions do not have the potential to be healed. On the other hand, an acorn swallowed by a pig would still have the potential to develop into an oak tree, since we could intervene, remove the acorn, and transplant it to a more conducive environment.[12] We might have good reasons for choosing not to remove the acorn, but the acorn still has the potential for becoming an oak tree. It has this potential in a more remote sense than that of an acorn already planted in the earth, but not as remote as that of an acorn becoming a pine tree, which is completely out of our hands. The same would apply to a patient whose condition could realistically be improved, even though the means might not be readily available. In some sense, it would be up to us whether we supplied those means

In contrast to Aristotle, who rules out certain potentials precisely because of some internal or external privation, Shewmon invokes the most remote and promiscuous sense of *potentiality*. For, if we acknowledge that an artificially sustained, brain-dead, or even decapitated human body has the potential for consciousness and other cognitive functions, then how can we rule out attributing this potential to all sorts of other things? Why can't we say, for example, that the vitality present in other species contains such potential? Indeed, does the possibility of altering the genes of some nonhuman animal to make that animal conscious and rational seem any more remote than the possibility of restoring consciousness to an artificially sustained, decapitated human body? Why is "vitality" even necessary? Why wouldn't a non-heart-beating cadaver qualify? Paraphrasing Shewmon, if bodies could be reconstituted and brought back to life, such as through implanted, futuristically transformed cells, then, theoretically, a dead person could be made to regain consciousness and other human functions.

Some might object that I have misconstrued Shewmon's position. Instead of relying on a notion of potentiality that is tied to material conditions and realistic probability, Shewmon may be invoking the notion of a spiritual soul as what gives life to the body. Such a soul, it may be claimed, has a radical power or potency for intellect and will that is unaffected by physiological changes such as the loss of a brain or decapitation. As long as the soul informs and animates the body, the potential (radical capacity or power) for intellect and will is present. Even if there were no conceivable technological way to restore brain function, the individual would still be alive as long as organic integration remained. Moreover, it might be claimed that, unless a being has a human soul, it could not have the functions of intellect and will. It may also be suggested that the potencies or powers an organism has are determined by the kind of organism it is. Thus, since a human being that has lost all brain function may still be considered a living member of the human species, as long as it retains circulatory and respiratory functions, then it remains "ensouled" with the power for intellect and will.

What sense there is to a "power" in an organism that is not tied to any notion of realistic possibility or physical conditions in the world is unclear. Not only would such a power have to be immaterial or spiritual, but there would be no rational basis for determining when such a radical power or potency for intellect and will is present in a thing. For example, why should we think that the power remains in an artificially sustained, brain-dead or decapitated human body as opposed to thinking that the power has left the body at this point? In Shewmon's earlier work, he accepted the Thomistic idea that matter must be disposed in a certain way to be ensouled. Powers were thereby linked to physical conditions, providing a more principled and reasonable way of determining whether and how a power could be present.[13] Moreover, if circulatory and respiratory functions provide sufficient evidence for the potential for intellect and will, then as long as those functions are maintained, regardless of any other changes the organism might undergo—such as more and more dismemberment so that all that remained was enough of the torso and internal organs for some artificially maintained circulatory and respiratory functions—such a body would have to be treated as a person and a being worthy of the highest moral standing. This is vitalism run amok.

To further illustrate why there is no rational basis for determining when such a radical power or potency for intellect and will is present in a thing, consider why there would be more reason for attributing it to a brain-dead human body than to, say, some living nonhuman animals, a living human cell that can undergo cloning, or a human cadaver in which rigor mortis has set in. Presumably Shewmon would not claim that these other beings have a human soul, so their ever developing intellect and will would, in his view, be inconceivable. The possibility that such beings could develop intellect and will, however, cannot be ruled out on conceptual grounds alone. Thus, the notion of such a radical power or potency is *conceptually* problematic. This also shows why we cannot link potentialities to kinds on conceptual grounds alone. Which potentialities or powers an organism has are tied to physical conditions in the organism and the world.

There are other conceptual difficulties in determining potentialities on the basis of species membership. Feldman (1992, 89–105) has suggested that we should regard dead specimens as belonging to their respective species; for example, butterflies carefully mounted are members of their respective species. After all, what else are they? Assuming that all members of the human species have the potential for intellect and will, however, would commit us to counting Jeremy Bentham and the pharaohs (perhaps more completely preserved) as human beings with the potential for intellect and will (cf. Wiggins 1980, 162; see my discussion in chapter 4). Even if we reject Feldman's suggestion and believe that an organism must be alive to count as a member of a species, we have the problem of determining when a member of a species ceases to be a member of that species. The obvious answer is that this occurs at death, that death is a change in kind of substance. Since the definition and criteria of death are precisely what are at issue, however, this reply does not help. Even if an artificially sustained, brain-dead human body and the hypothetically sustained, decapitated human body are living organisms, are they living members of the human species, as opposed to the remains of a living member of the human species, or a member of some other kind of thing? By artificially sustaining brain-dead human bodies or, hypothetically, decapitated human bodies, we intervene in the life history of the organism in such a radical way that we create new kinds of beings, and we should recognize that the human being or "person" has died. Thus, even if the potential for intellect and will were linked to membership in the human species, it is questionable whether such artificially sustained bodies should be treated as members of that species.[14]

In conclusion, if potentiality comes in degrees, as I have argued, then we need to ask which sense of potentiality is relevant to the task of defining death. The remote or conceptually problematic sense that Shewmon invokes seems to be, as Feinberg says, "so promiscuous" as to be of little use. Indeed, since the matter of defining death is in part an ethical task, we should perhaps follow Aristotle's advice (*Nicomachean Ethics* 1.3.1094b11–15) to not seek more precision than the subject matter admits and acknowledge that we are in the realm of probabilities, rather than certainties. In fact, the burden of proof should rest on those who wish to deny the significance of the realistic probabilities that are involved in assessing which potentialities are real.[15]

Although the concept of potentiality is notoriously difficult, there have been attempts to try to articulate this more proximate and more sensible notion of potentiality (Covey 1991; Kottow 1984; Annis 1984; Ray 1985), usually by specifying some condition, such as a high degree of probability that the potential will be actualized, that the potential will be actualized in the "natural or normal course of events," or that unusual circumstances will not intervene to prevent the potential from being realized. Regardless of whether any of these attempts have been successful, the remote kind of potentiality that Shewmon considers lacks any and all of these conditions. The "brain-dead" human being certainly will not regain consciousness "in the natural course of events." In fact, artificially sustaining a brain-dead body falls outside the natural or normal course of events. It is more a technological artifact. The brain-dead body is not disposed to regain consciousness if nothing unusual intervenes, and the probability of its regaining consciousness is extremely low. Thus, not only is Aristotle's account of potentiality inapplicable, but none of these modern accounts of potentiality is compatible with attributing the potential for consciousness to a human being whose brain has been destroyed.[16]

On the basis of a more sensible, Aristotelian concept of potentiality, Shewmon drew the correct conclusions in his 1985 article: acceptance of a consciousness-related formulation of death coheres best with a substantive view of personhood. This view recognizes that the potential for consciousness is necessary for personhood and that a particular biological substrate, more than simply being a specimen of the human species, is necessary for that potential. This view is consistent not only with the current neurological criterion for death—loss of all brain functions, including the brainstem—but with a consciousness-related criterion as well.

Note that the view that a particular biological substrate, more than simply being a specimen of the human species, is necessary for the potential for consciousness is consistent with the position taken by some (though perhaps not most) Catholic scholars. This is perhaps most clearly seen in a report by a bioethics section of the International Federation of Catholic Universities that met from December 1987 to June 1988 to study the question of anencephaly. The report stated, as quoted by a Catholic Bishop at the Eighth Bishops' Workshop in Dallas, Texas, in 1989:

> In cases of established anencephaly, the following considerations apply:
>
> 1. We do not claim to know or to study here the full essential requirements for being a person. That remains an important and still open ethical and legal question. But the enjoyment of moral protections provided to those thought to be persons demands a minimal biological substrate as a basis for future development.
> 2. In the absence of biological conditions for the possibility of any capacity for future relationships or self-consciousness, there is either no human person or no longer a human person.
> 3. Therefore, those who advise or choose to terminate a pregnancy in which anencephaly has been clearly established cannot be said to be acting in a way that is morally wrong unless on other grounds.
> 4. Furthermore, the use of anencephalics after delivery as the source of organ or tissue retrieval is not a violation of personal dignity. Therefore, if such retrieval is considered morally wrong, it must be on other grounds. (R. Smith 1989, 275–76)[17]

The details of the theological justification for this view do not appear in the proceedings of the Bishops' Workshop, but William Wallace, O.P., has argued that St. Thomas Aquinas accepted the possibility that "the human soul may depart from the body before all signs of life have disappeared from it" (Wallace 1995, 394). Wallace notes that Aquinas is widely known for his view of "delayed hominization," his teaching that "the beginning of life is a gradual process, that the human soul is not infused into the incipient organism at fertilization but rather is prepared for by a succession of forms that dispose the matter for the reception of a rational soul"; but, Wallace observes, "little attention has been paid to the obverse of that process, what might be termed 'early dehominization,' where the human soul departs from the body at some period of time before all bodily functions have ceased" (394, 397).

Wallace notes that, although Aquinas did not develop his thought on this subject, his commentary on Proposition 1 of the *Liber de causis* recognizes the possibility of the reversal of delayed hominization. In this work, Aquinas states, "For it is obvious that in the generation of an individual human being one finds in the material subject first existence, then the living thing and after that a human: for it is an animal before it is a man, as is said in the second book of *On the Generation of Animals*. And again, in the process of corruption, first [the individual] loses the use of reason and remains alive and breathing, then it loses life and remains a being, because it does not corrupt into nothingness" (Aquinas *Super librum de causis expositio*, quoted in Wallace 1995, 397).

In applying this interpretation of Aquinas to the contemporary problem of defining death, Wallace suggests that Aquinas's view supports the position that Shewmon took in his early work in 1985. As noted above, Shewmon then held that the human person dies and the rational soul departs when there is irreversible destruction of the part of the brain necessary for the functioning of intellect and will, even if the human organism or "humanoid" continues to live. Wallace also cites the analysis of human death and dying offered by Mieczysaw A. Krpiec, O.P. (1985), as cohering with Aquinas's view of "delayed dehominization":

> In discussing the death of a human person, Krpiec makes a distinction between the cessation of life signs when the soul is thought to leave the body, which he calls "physical death," and death "understood actively," that is, death as a real experience of the human spirit. The latter experience occurs at the moment when the person becomes capable of making a final decision about life, a moment that represents the culmination of all the changeable acts performed during the entire span of bodily existence. Active death, Krpiec argues, is the transtemporal experience that takes place in the realm of the spirit and beyond the point at which the individual can return to the temporal and changeable condition of earthly life. Thus, it does not coincide with the co-activity of the body. The implication is that the human soul at the moment of active death has already departed from the body and subsists as an individual substance. (Wallace 1995, 405)

In pointing out that there may be some theological justification in the Catholic tradition for rejecting a species view of person and accepting a consciousness-related definition and criterion of death, I am not suggesting that this is the *only* interpretation within that tradition.[18] My point is simply to show that the species view of persons fails to cohere with at least some interpretations of the notion of person in the

Catholic tradition and that a consciousness-related definition and criterion of death is consistent with and may be entailed by certain interpretations within that tradition. I have also offered reasons for why I think the notion of potentiality that some, like Shewmon, invoke is useless and cannot serve as a basis for a reasonable view about persons and death. My critical discussion is offered as a contribution to what needs to be a much more robust discussion within the Catholic tradition, as well as others, about the meaning of death. It is important for members of all religious denominations and philosophical persuasions to examine their traditions in the light of challenges posed by advances in medical technology. The clinical cases are new. They pose unprecedented challenges to our religious, philosophical, moral, and cultural systems of beliefs. Instead of blindly accepting a medical opinion about what death is and when it occurs, we should examine our systems of belief and engage in critical discourse with those in and outside our own traditions. To fail to do so is to act in bad faith. It is to abdicate our responsibility to determine who we are.

CHAPTER SEVEN

Persons as Qualities or Phases of Human Organisms

The constitutive interpretation of the relation between the person and the human being explains how there can be a divergence in the life histories of persons and human beings and how, at the same time, a person can be a substance without generating a case of relative identity. It may be claimed, however, that we should abandon the notion that persons are substances in favor of treating them as phases or functional specifications of some other substance (e.g., human beings). As noted in earlier chapters, the biological paradigm of death assumes this view of persons.

Examples of phased predicates, or "phased sortals," include *infant, adult, tadpole, caterpillar, pupa, banker, mayor,* and *sapling.* These predicates apply during certain points in the life history of whatever substance they restrict. Substance concepts, or "substance sortals," such as *human being, horse,* and *tree,* are distinguished from phased predicates in that they (1) answer in a fundamental sense what something is and (2) apply throughout an individual's life history. Thus, *boy* and *mayor* are phased predicates, because the individual referred to by, say, the boy John Doe or the mayor John Doe may continue to exist even though that individual is no longer a boy or no longer a mayor. Substance concepts, in contrast, entail the individual ceasing to exist if it no longer satisfies the concept. Thus, if *person* is a genuine substance concept for John Doe, then if John Doe ceases to be a person, John Doe ceases to exist.[1]

Since the biological paradigm of death treats *person* as a phased sortal concept, Bernat, Culver, and Gert (1982a, 1982b; Bernat 1998; Culver and Gert 1982) hold that, even though the person, for example, Nancy Cruzan, may no longer exist when she has irreversibly lost consciousness, this does not mean that Nancy

Cruzan necessarily ceases to exist. The organism has simply lost some set of non-essential qualities that we group together as the referent of *person*. Just as *banker* denotes a set of qualities or functions that bankers typically engage in and that define the profession, so, too, *person* denotes a set of qualities or functions that human beings (and perhaps members of other species, such as apes, dolphins, or creatures on some distant planet) typically engage in and that define personhood. The biological paradigm treats *human being* or *human organism* as the substance concept of which personhood is a phase. Thus, only when Nancy Cruzan ceases to be a human organism does Nancy Cruzan cease to exist. In this view, *person* is treated like other phased sortals, such as *banker* or *boy*. Even though a banker leaves her job or a boy grows up to be a man, this does not entail these individuals ceasing to exist. The banker and boy may no longer exist, but the human being that was the banker or boy does. As Bernat, Culver, and Gert maintain, phases are not the kind of thing that literally dies.

The phased sortal interpretation of person would enable us to interpret the cases of total amnesia and permanent vegetative state (PermVS) as cases in which a person ceases to exist (i.e., the person phase ends) without the individual (i.e., the organism) ceasing to exist. Also, in the case of total amnesia, it could be maintained under the phased sortal interpretation that a new person starts to exist. Thus, with respect to Locke's memory criterion of personal identity, the phased sortal interpretation enables us to countenance the possibility of two or more persons sharing one body. Since the person is identified with a set of abilities and qualities—that is, a certain functional specification—and since the sets of abilities and qualities are so different before and after the amnesia, the phased sortal interpretation would likely treat the radically disconnected sets of memories and mental qualities as different persons. Note that the constitutive interpretation, in contrast, can appeal to the essential matter underlying the psychological functions in support of treating the total amnesiac as the same person. The matter underlying the phase, however, is irrelevant in a view that treats the person simply as a set of qualities or functions.

This reasoning underlies Locke's treatment of the hypothetical case of body swapping: "For should the Soul of a Prince, carrying with it the consciousness of the Prince's past life, enter and inform the Body of a Cobler as soon as deserted by his own Soul, every one sees, he would be the same Person with the Prince, accountable only for the Prince's actions: But who would say it was the same Man?" (Locke [1694] 1975, 340). In Locke's view, the person is a set of interconnected mental properties that extend through time in the form of memory. While Locke assumes that consciousness and memory inhere in some type of substance, the substance that underlies the consciousness and memories is irrelevant to personal identity:

> *Self* is that conscious thinking thing, (whatever Substance, made up of whether Spiritual, or Material, Simple, or Compounded, it matters not), which is sensible, or conscious of Pleasure and Pain, capable of Happiness or Misery, and so is concern'd for it *self*, as far as that consciousness extends. Thus every one finds, that whilst comprehended under that consciousness, the little Finger is as much a part of it *self*, as what is most so. Upon separation of this little Finger, should this consciousness go along with the little Finger, and leave the rest of the Body, 'tis evident the little Finger would be the *Person*, the same *Person*; and *self* then would have nothing to do with the rest of the Body. As in this case it is the consciousness that goes along with the Substance, when one part is separated from the other, which makes the same Person, and constitutes this inseparable *self*: so it is in reference to Substances remote in time. That with which the *consciousness* of this present thinking thing can join it self, makes the same *Person*, and is one *self* with it, and with nothing else; and so attributes to it *self*, and owns all the Actions of that thing, as its own, as far as that consciousness reaches, and no farther; as every one who reflects will perceive. (341)

Locke's view of consciousness and the person is the inspiration for contemporary functionalist theories of the mind, since, in this view, what makes a mind is functionality, rather than any substance that underlies the function. The functionalist theory holds that minds can be realized in a variety of substances, including not just the biological organisms that we are most familiar with but, conceivably, sophisticated computers and (some even countenance) immaterial souls. Locke's view of personal identity led to David Hume's "bundle" theory in which a person is just a bundle of interrelated psychological properties: there is no person or self as a substantive being of any kind (Hume [1739] 1978, 251–63). It is also the inspiration for Derek Parfit's influential contemporary view of persons.

Like the constitutive interpretation of the relation between the person and the human organism, the phased sortal interpretation provides a way to distinguish the person from the human organism without violating the constraints of the absoluteness of identity. It enables us to say, P: Nancy Cruzan, the person who was in the automobile accident, is the *same human organism* as Nancy Cruzan in the hospital bed following her accident, but not the *same person* (for Nancy Cruzan in a PermVS after the accident is not a person). This may seem to be a case of relative identity—that is, a case in which *a* is the same F (human organism) as *b*, and *a* is a G (person), but *a* is not the same G (person) as *b*. If *person* is a phased sortal and not a substance sortal, however, we can use Wiggins's explanation of "type-(3)" purported cases of relative identity to show why P is not a genuine case of relative identity.[2] Thus, if both the constitutive and phased sortal interpretations respect the absoluteness of identity, then the choice between these interpretations will depend on considerations other than whether one or the other violates the absoluteness of identity.

Many arguments have been advanced for and against the qualitative Lockean/ Parfitian view of persons. It is beyond the scope of this work to deal with all of them, but, given that the issue is ultimately critical to the definition of death, I address here some of these arguments and raise what I think are the most serious objections to the view. I begin with some general remarks on the violence done to our language if we accept persons as phases of human organisms, and then consider some of the thought experiments that Locke and Parfit offer in support of their views. When we take into consideration the importance of the first-person perspective and the moral and cultural dimensions of persons, the thought experiments fail to yield the intuitive results that Locke and Parfit have claimed for them. In fact, there is a methodological problem with Parfit's thought experiments involving replication: these thought experiments sunder persons from their moral and cultural context. Since persons and personal identity are in part determined by moral and cultural factors, there is no way to evaluate our intuitions about the hypothetical cases involving replication without some knowledge of what the moral and cultural context would be in an age of replication.

I also review the criticism originally leveled by Bishop Butler and Thomas Reid against Locke's view that any psychological criterion of personal identity, such as Locke's memory criterion, is bound to be circular and must *presuppose* personal identity. This criticism continues to plague contemporary versions of the theory, such as those of H. P. Grice ([1941] 1975) and Derek Parfit (1986). In addition, P. F. Strawson's argument that persons are primitive entities and that mental states cannot be individuated or identified without reference to them continues to hold true. Butler's and Reid's criticism and Strawson's view argue against treating persons as phases of some other substance, such as a human organism.

VIOLENCE TO LANGUAGE

In chapter 3, I pointed out that a kind of violence would be done to our linguistic practice if we were to accept Bernat, Culver, and Gert's treatment of persons as phases rather than substances. In their view, *death* cannot be applied literally to persons because *death* is a biological concept appropriate to human organisms, not to roles, functions, abilities, or qualities of awareness. Many of us, however, commonly predicate terms such as *death, living, breathing, eating,* and *sleeping* to persons and do not think there is anything metaphorical about doing so. Our talk assumes that persons are substantive entities, not phases. We regard personal identity as consisting of the persistence of a substantive being, rather than a relation between various phases of some other kind of being that may or may not persist.[3] To accept the idea that persons are phases of human organisms, we would have to give up this linguistic practice of literally predicating such familiar terms to persons.

Proponents of the whole-brain formulation of death, such as Bernat, Culver, and Gert, have maintained that their view, in contrast to the consciousness-related formulation, captures what *death* means in the nontechnical way traditionally used by the public. For example, James Bernat criticizes the consciousness-related formulation because it is "not what society means by death" (Bernat 1998, 17). He can sustain this claim, however, only by maintaining that persons do not literally die, which conflicts with the way in which many people have traditionally spoken about persons and their death. While the divergence of Bernat, Culver, and Gert's understanding of person from the traditional and ordinary understanding of persons as substantive entities certainly does not mean error, this shows what is at stake in terms of conceptual and linguistic revision if we accept their view. Moreover, since these authors have claimed that their view accords with the traditional and nontechnical understanding of *death* among the general public and have argued that this agreement provides support for the acceptability of their view, it is important to show how their proposal conflicts with the traditional understanding of *person* as a kind of thing that can literally die. Whereas the general public and many philosophers have predicated death to persons, Bernat, Culver, and Gert assume that such predication is conceptually impossible and that the public and these philosophers have been speaking metaphorically all along.

LOCKE'S THOUGHT EXPERIMENTS

Locke rejected the idea that a person can be identified with any substance, material or immaterial. According to Locke, "consciousness alone makes self." He considers the possibility of transmigration of the soul in reincarnation and says that there is no way to know how many souls may be associated with a single person but that this does not affect our judgment of personal identity. He also considers the possibility of "two distinct incommunicable consciousnesses acting in the same Body, the one constantly by Day, the other by Night; and on the other side the same consciousness acting by Intervals two distinct Bodies" (Locke [1694] 1975, 344). He rhetorically asks, "in the first case, Whether the *Day* and the *Night-man* would not be two as distinct Persons, as *Socrates* and *Plato*; and whether in the second case, there would not be one Person in two distinct Bodies, as much as one Man is the same in two distinct clothings." "Nor is it at all material to say," Locke continues, "that this same, and this distinct *consciousness* in the cases above-mentioned, is owing to the same and distinct immaterial Substances, bringing it with them to those Bodies, which whether true or no, alters not the case: Since 'tis evident the *personal Identity* would equally be determined by the consciousness, whether that consciousness were annexed to some individual Substance or no." He concludes, "*self* is not determined by Identity or Diversity of Substance, which it cannot be sure of, but only by Identity of consciousness" (344–45).

Descartes thought that he could have a direct awareness or intuition of himself as a thinking, nonextended, indivisible substance, but Locke's empiricism committed him to the belief that we could not have any awareness or knowledge of substance, material or immaterial. Locke also thought that this did not affect our judgments of personal identity, because consciousness alone, insofar as it extends through time, was a sufficient criterion for personal identity. What made it sufficient was that he believed it provided the most sensible answers to the kinds of questions we ask about persons and their identity. For Locke, these questions were in the moral and legal domain. Thus, Locke states that *person* is "a Forensick term appropriating Actions and their Merit; and so belongs only to intelligent Agents, capable of Law, and Happiness and Misery" (346).

Thus, of the three aspects that Wiggins says we try to hold in a single focus in our concept of person, Locke recognized only two: the importance of consciousness and the central role of the concept of person in our moral and legal thought. Since Locke conceives of persons as independent of the substance that underlies consciousness, persons are not treated as objects of biological, anatomical, and neurophysiological inquiry. Ultimately, I shall argue, the problem for Locke's account of person, and for the accounts of those who have followed his lead in advocating a qualitative rather than substantive view of persons (e.g., Derek Parfit), is that such a view fails to provide a sensible foundation for our moral and legal thought about persons. As a forensic term, the qualitative view of persons falls short because it ignores the importance assigned to our biological nature in our moral and legal thought.

Because Locke linked moral responsibility with personal identity, his views about moral responsibility and personal identity were interdependent. His considerations of moral responsibility provided support for his memory criterion of personal identity, while his memory criterion provided support for his views about moral responsibility. Thus, in considering cases that raised the issue of moral responsibility, Locke concluded that a person could be held responsible only for those actions that he or she remembered doing. For example, in cases such as the Jekyll/Hyde scenario described in chapter 5, in which the person by day does not have the same consciousness as the person by night, Locke would conclude that it would be wrong to hold the person by day responsible for what was done by the person by night, and vice versa. In the case of someone who forgets a part or all of his life, Locke also concluded that it would be wrong to hold the person responsible for past actions that the person has no recollection of doing. In the case of the somnambulist who unconsciously commits some act while sleepwalking, the waking person cannot be held responsible for the act. Finally, Locke considers whether someone should be punished for heinous acts committed while drunk, if, while drunk, the person was not conscious of doing those acts. Locke again draws the logical implication of his memory criterion of personal identity: the law would justly punish this individual, but only because the law cannot determine the truth of the individual's plea of not being conscious while drunk. If the person were really not conscious of his actions while drunk, then there would be no basis, according to Locke, for holding him responsible for those acts. Locke concludes his discussion of this case, "But, in the great Day, wherein the Secrets of all Hearts shall be laid open, it may be reasonable to think, no one shall be made to answer for what he knows nothing of; but shall receive his Doom, his Conscience accusing or excusing him" (344).

Soon after Locke wrote *An Essay Concerning Human Understanding*, he was met with a barrage of criticism by some of the most formidable thinkers of his day, including Leibniz, Hume, Butler, Reid, and his friend Molyneux. Molyneux distinguished the case of the somnambulist from that of the drunkard and argued that, while the somnambulist is not responsible for his condition, drunkenness is a voluntarily induced state and the drunkard should therefore be held accountable for his actions while drunk. Henry Allison (1966, 46) points out that Locke ultimately admitted that the drunkard is justifiably punished for his crimes, even though he is not conscious of them. This admission that moral responsibility may extend beyond what one remembers about one's acts is significant because it shows the inadequacy of the memory criterion of personal identity for our moral thinking about persons.

Similar problems for Locke's view were raised by Berkeley, Reid, and Leibniz. Reid asked, "Suppose a brave officer to have been flogged when a boy at school, for robbing an orchard, to have taken a standard for the enemy in his first campaign, and to have been made a general in advanced life. Suppose also, which must be admitted to be possible, that when he took the standard he was conscious of his having been flogged at school, and that when made a general he was conscious of his taking the standard, but had absolutely lost consciousness of his flogging" (Reid [1895] 1969, 352). Locke's memory criterion of personal identity would commit him to identifying the boy with the person who took the standard, and the person who took the standard with the general. But, because the general has no memory of the flogging, the general cannot be the same person as the boy. This generates a contradiction, since the transitivity of identity entails the general being identical to the boy.

Modern psychological continuity theorists of personal identity have suggested that Locke's memory criterion can be modified in a way that obviates this specific objection. Thus, Grice ([1941] 1975) proposes that *a* is the same person as *b* as long as there is an overlapping chain of memories that link *a* and *b*. For example, as long as the officer remembers being flogged as a boy and the general remembers the officer's first campaign, the general and the boy are psychologically linked through overlapping memories, even though the general has no memory of being flogged as a boy.[4]

Several difficulties persist with this proposal. I discuss the first two immediately below, then consider additional problems after presenting Parfit's further modifications and extension of the Lockean view. First, Grice's proposal does not explain how we may continue to exist despite periods of unconsciousness. Few memories link our unconscious states with our conscious ones (recollecting our dreams is one exception), thus it is unclear whether the memory criterion can account for how a person may persist through periods of unconsciousness. Technically, since our unconscious states are not part of the chain of overlapping memories, they cannot be identified as belonging to the person. If we think persons persist through periods of unconsciousness and that those unconscious states are states of the person, then personal identity must consist in something more than overlapping chains of memories.[5]

Second, the modification to Locke's criterion does not account for amnesia, where amnesia may break the chain of memories. This was Leibniz's concern:

> Neither would I say that personal identity and even the self do not dwell in us and that I am not this ego which has been in the cradle, under pretext that I no more remember anything of all that I then did. It is sufficient in order to find moral identity by itself that there be a *middle bond of consciousness* between a state bordering upon or even a little removed from another, although a leap or forgotten interval might be mingled therein. Thus if a disease had caused an interruption of the continuity of the bond of consciousness so that I did not know how I came into the present state, although I remember things more remote, the testimony of others could fill the void in my memory. I could even be punished upon this testimony, if I had just done something bad of deliberate purpose in an interval that I had forgotten a little after on account of this disease. And if I had just forgotten all past things and would be obliged to let myself be taught anew even to my name and even to reading and writing, I could always learn

from others my past life in my previous state, as I have kept my rights without its being necessary for me to share them with two persons, and to make me the heir of myself. (Leibniz [1690] 1981, paras. 236–37)[6]

Commenting on the passage from Leibniz, Allison points out,

> Here we see the discussion carried out on an ethical and legal level, divorced from any metaphysical considerations, and the clear result is that there are important instances where moral responsibility must be extended beyond memory. Not explicit awareness, Leibniz argues, but merely "a middle bond of consciousness" (*une moyenne liason de consciosité*) between two distinct states is enough to establish it is identity, and hence, the accountability of the person. Even if an individual suffers a temporary loss of memory, so that he cannot recall the immediate past, the testimony of others is sufficient to establish the necessary unifying bond, and the individual should not only regard himself as the author of the deeds attributed to him. (Allison 1966, 54)

Leibniz's commentary is significant because it suggests that personal identity is not simply determined by some internal connection among our psychological states but is in part determined by how others regard us. Because someone who suffers amnesia is treated in many moral and legal respects as the same person, the metaphysical considerations for treating the amnesiac as a different person—that is, the amnesiac's failure to meet the psychological continuity criterion of personal identity— must be rejected. An alternative metaphysical account must therefore be given to accord with our moral intuitions. The constitutive interpretation is such an account, since it treats sameness of human organism as a necessary condition for personal identity, allows for social and cultural factors to determine, in part, personal identity, and maintains that the same first-person perspective would persist through cases of total amnesia.

A basic difficulty for the Lockean account is that it is too narrow. By focusing on conscious states and memory relations between those states, Locke ignores other aspects of personhood that are relevant to our moral and legal thought about persons. The details are important. In some cases, moral considerations may weigh in as justification for our claims about personal identity, as in Molyneux's explanation of why the drunkard's loss of consciousness of what he did while drunk does not justify treating him as a different person when he becomes sober. In the case of the somnambulist, the moral considerations argue against holding him responsible for his actions while asleep, but they do not justify treating him as a different person from the person when awake. Although the memory criterion along with considerations about moral responsibility argue for treating the person when asleep as different from the person when awake, other considerations—such as a more general psy-chological theory that links conscious and unconscious states or legal considerations regarding ownership of property that do not dissipate when one falls asleep—argue in favor of treating them as the same person. Leibniz's observation that the amne-siac would not lose his property, rights, and so forth, is an example of how moral and legal considerations bear on our judgments of personal identity.

PARFIT'S VIEW

In recent times, Derek Parfit (1986) has modified the Lockean memory criterion of personal identity to one of psychological continuity. In response to Reid's type of objection to Locke's view, Parfit endorses Grice's suggestion of an overlapping chain of memories, but he also allows overlapping connections between psychological states other than memory to constitute psychological continuity over time—for ex-ample, connections between past desires and present intentions, stable personality traits, habits, beliefs, and abilities. If more than half of these psychological connec-tions hold between a and b over time, then, Parfit says, a is "strongly psychologically connected" to b. In other words, if b on Tuesday has at least half of the memories, personality traits, desires, and so forth as a had on Monday, then there is strong psy-chological connectedness between a and b. Psychological connectedness thus comes in degrees. "Psychological continuity" is made up of overlapping chains of strong psychological connectedness (Parfit 1986, 206). Thus, psychological conti-nuity between a at t_1 and c at t_3 does not require a strong psychological connected-ness between a and c. As long as a at t_1 is strongly psychologically connected to b at t_2, and b at t_2 is strongly psychologically connected to c at t_3, then a and c are psy-chologically continuous.

Psychological continuity is necessary, but not sufficient, for personal identity. In order for a to be the same person as b, Parfit adds two further conditions: the psy-chological continuity (1) must have the right kind of cause and (2) must not have taken a branching form. These conditions are necessary, according to Parfit, be-cause we can conceive of cases in which the normal causal connections for psy-chological continuity, such as the persistence of the same physical body or brain over time, may not obtain and yet there may be psychological continuity. In addi-tion, the causal connections can take a branching form. According to Parfit, such a scenario would take place in the following hypothetical case:

> I enter the Teletransporter. I have been to Mars before, but only by the old method, a
> space-ship journey taking several weeks. This machine will send me at the speed of

light. I merely have to press the green button. Like others, I am nervous. Will it work? I remind myself what I have been told to expect. When I press the button, I shall lose consciousness, and then wake up at what seems a moment later. In fact I shall have been unconscious for about an hour. The Scanner here on Earth will destroy my brain and body, while recording the exact states of all of my cells. It will then transmit this information by radio. Traveling at the speed of light, the message will take three minutes to reach the Replicator on Mars. This will then create, out of new matter, a brain and body exactly like mine. It will be in this body that I shall wake up.

Though I believe that this is what will happen, I still hesitate. But then I remember seeing my wife grin when, at breakfast today, I revealed my nervousness. As she reminded me, she has been often teletransported, and there is nothing wrong with *her*. I press the button. As predicted, I lose and seem at once to regain consciousness, but in a different cubicle. Examining my new body, I find no change at all. Even the cut on my upper lip, from this morning's shave, is still there.

Several years pass, during which I am often Teletransported. I am now back in the cubicle, ready for another trip to Mars. But this time, when I press the green button, I do not lose consciousness. There is a whirring sound, then silence. I leave the cubicle, and say to the attendant: "It's not working. What did I do wrong?"

"It's working," he replies, handing me a printed card. This reads: "The New Scanner records your blueprint without destroying your brain and body. We hope that you will welcome the opportunities which this technical advance offers."

The attendant tells me that I am one of the first people to use the New Scanner. He adds that, if I stay for an hour, I can use the intercom to see and talk to myself on Mars.

"Wait a minute," I reply, "If I am here I can't *also* be on Mars."

Someone politely coughs, a white-coated man who asks to speak to me in private. We go to his office, where he tells me to sit down, and pauses. Then he says: "I'm afraid that we're having problems with the New Scanner. It records your blueprint just as accurately, as you will see when you talk to yourself on Mars. But it seems to be damaging the cardiac systems which it scans. Judging from the results so far, though you will be quite healthy on Mars, here on Earth you must expect cardiac failure within the next few days."

The attendant calls me to the Intercom. On the screen I see myself just as I do in the mirror every morning. But there are two differences. On the screen I am not left-right reversed. And while I stand here speechless, I can see and hear myself, in the studio on Mars, starting to speak. (Parfit 1986, 200–201)

Parfit claims that, because consideration of such imaginary cases arouses strong beliefs in us about ourselves, "we discover what we believe to be involved in our own continued existence, or what it is that makes us now and ourselves next year the same people" (201). He claims that, when we consider the scenario above, we are strongly inclined to believe we would continue to exist through teletransportation or that at least anything that is important to us about our identity would be preserved through teletransportation.[7] What is preserved is psychological continuity without bodily continuity.

The malfunction in the teletransporter creates a puzzling situation. The person who steps out of the teletransporter on Earth is also psychologically continuous with the person who stepped into the teletransporter, so we would also be inclined to say that these persons are identical. If psychological continuity were sufficient for personal identity, we would then have to identify the person who steps into the teletransporter with both the person on Mars and the person on Earth. Since identity is transitive, we would have to identify the person on Mars with the person on Earth. But a single person cannot exist in two places at once. Thus, Parfit concludes that psychological continuity is necessary but insufficient for personal identity. What happens in the branching case of teletransportation, according to Parfit, is that the person who steps into the teletransporter *survives* in two different locations; because survival is not a transitive relation, there is no contradiction in holding that a person can survive in more than one place at a time. Parfit's criterion of personal identity thus requires that psychological continuity must take place with the normal, non-branching cause.

What is most radical and Lockean in spirit about Parfit's view is his proposal that "what really matters" to us is our survival, not our identity. In the branching case, Parfit takes comfort in the fact that there is someone on Mars who has the same beliefs, desires, projects, memories, and so on. The continuation of his psychology, he claims, is all that he rationally and prudentially is concerned about when it comes to his survival. What difference does it make if his psychology happens to be realized in other matter or in more than one place? K. T. Maslin observes, "the Locke/Parfit approach is analogous to treating you as a function or program run on the hardware of the brain, the material embodiment being strictly irrelevant to your identity and survival. You could go from body and brain to body and brain, just as information on a floppy disc can be transferred intact to another disc if the original becomes damaged" (Maslin 2001, 275).

Parfit claims that the beliefs aroused by the fictional cases should cohere with one's theory about the relation of mind and body: "When we ask what persons are and how they continue to exist, the fundamental question is a choice between two views. On one view, we are separately existing entities, distinct from our brains and bodies and our experience, and entities whose existence must be all-or-nothing. The other view is the Reductionist View. And I claim that, of these, the second view is true" (Parfit 1986, 273). Thus, one may believe identity rather than survival is what matters only if one believes in the existence of Cartesian egos (265–66). Once one accepts reductionism or the view that personal identity consists in physical and/or psychological continuity and that it can hold as a matter of degree, Parfit believes, one should accept the conclusion that survival or relation R (psychological continuity) is all that matters.[8]

Another way of stating Parfit's view is that he takes the belief (1) that we are separately existing entities distinct from our brains, bodies, and experiences as necessary for the beliefs (2) that our existence must always be determinate and (3) that identity rather than survival is what matters. Parfit understands the belief that we are separately existing entities as tantamount to a belief in Cartesian egos: immaterial minds, souls, or spiritual substances. In addition, he believes that, if one rejects Cartesian egos, one must accept reductionism. Then, once one accepts reductionism and considers what to say about cases such as the "Combined Spectrum" (another hypothetical case, discussed later in the chapter), one should conclude that our continued existence may be indeterminate and a matter of degree. Again, personal survival—the continuation of our psychological continuity rather than our personal identity—is "what fundamentally matters" (Parfit 1986, 217).

Parfit admits that there is another nonreductionist view, which holds that, although we are not separately existing entities, separate from our brains, bodies, and experiences, personal identity is a further fact beyond just physical and/or psychological continuity. He calls this the "Further Fact View." He dismisses this view. In his discussion of the Combined Spectrum, he claims this view is indefensible because it fails to explain in what further fact personal identity is supposed to consist if not the fact that we are separately existing entities (240).

One can be justified, however, in holding beliefs (2) and (3) on grounds other than a belief in Cartesian egos. Rejecting the existence of Cartesian egos does not commit one to the view that personal identity can be indeterminate or a matter of degree. Nor does it commit one to the view that survival is all that matters. Moreover, rejection of the existence of Cartesian egos does not entail acceptance of Parfit's reductionism. For example, one can accept a nonreductive and supervenient, constitutive relation between the person and human organism and accept beliefs (2) and (3).[9] In this case, the "Further Fact" about personal identity would consist in the same person continuing to be constituted by the same human organism. Moreover, since the constitutive view treats relational properties as essential to persons, these properties are further facts about personal identity that need to be taken into account. This nonreductive, materialistic view of persons differs significantly from the Cartesian position. Nonreductive materialists understand persons as dependent on, though not reducible or identical to, material bodies.[10] Persons are distinct from human organisms but do not exist separately from them in the way a Cartesian mind is thought to exist separately from a material body. Cartesian dualists understand persons as capable of existing as immaterial substances. Also, Descartes claimed to have direct intuition of himself as a thinking thing. Materialists may reject such an intuition and, like Locke and Parfit, attempt to ground their account in empirical theory. Thus, Locke and Parfit may be right to reject some of the metaphysical excesses of Cartesianism, but their reasons for rejecting Cartesianism do not necessarily tell against other substantive views of persons. Indeed, in Parfit's case, he seems to ignore these other substantive views and presents his case as an either/or choice between Cartesianism and his Lockean-inspired alternative. Butler commits the same error of assuming that there are only two alternative positions. Although Butler's criticism of the circularity in the Lockean account is correct, it does not automatically lead to the Cartesian view, as Butler assumed. Instead, the metaphysical and moral arguments for and against the various views need to be considered with the aim of deciding which theory best accounts for our understanding of persons as biological, conscious, moral beings.

Parfit's view, no less than Locke's in his day, has generated a great deal of critical discussion. The point of departure for some of this criticism has been a discussion of the thought experiments that Parfit uses to support his claim that personal survival (i.e., psychological continuity) rather than personal identity is all that really matters to us. Some philosophers, including Michael Lockwood (1985, 1994), David Wiggins (1987, 2001), Peter Unger (1990), and Jeff McMahan (2002), have challenged the intuitions that Parfit claims to have about the thought experiments. In their view, consideration of Parfit's hypothetical cases, along with other cases, yields the intuition that continuity of our body or brain is a significant part of what matters to us.

Unger (1990) suggests that Parfit's "teletransporter" can be understood as a taping device that records the positions of your molecules and then takes new matter on Mars to construct a replica. But, Unger thinks, when understood in this way, the initial intuitive plausibility that one is "transported" to Mars fades. His intuition is that, once you press the green button and your brain and body are destroyed on Earth, you are destroyed. What happens to some other matter on Mars has nothing to do with whether you survive. He thinks we can continue to exist while undergoing the gradual replacement of bodily parts over time, but that this is not possible when replacement occurs in one go.

McMahan also challenges Parfit's intuitions about teletransportation with the following thought experiment:

> The Suicide Mission: In a time of war, one has been chosen to carry out a military mission that will involve certain death. Although the operation of the Replicator is very expensive and has therefore been strictly rationed, one's superiors have granted one the privilege of having a replica of oneself made prior to the mission. They will also allow one to choose, prior to the process of replication, whether one will go on the mission oneself or whether the replica will be sent. (Because one is a dutiful soldier, one's replica will be dutiful as well. One knows that if ordered, he will go on the mission.) (McMahan 2002, 57)

McMahan points out that most of us would, without hesitation, choose that our replica should be sent on the mission, but that this intuition conflicts with Parfit's: "Yet, according to the Psychological Account of Egoistic Concern, all that matters in the relation that the original person bears to himself in the future is also present in the relation that he will bear to his replica. On this view, it should make no difference to the person, prior to replication, whether it is he himself or his replica who will be sent on the mission" (McMahan 2002, 57).

A similar conflict in intuitions can be seen in the consideration of how one would receive the news from the teletransporter attendant about one's impending death on Earth caused by the New Scanner. Parfit thinks that talking to his replica on Mars would console him a little, especially if the replica promised to love his wife, care for his children, complete his projects, and so on. He would soon come to think that dying with a replica is not as bad as simply dying. In fact, although it may be natural to assume that one's prospects on Earth in the branch-line case are as bad as ordinary death, Parfit denies this. He argues that we "ought to regard having a Replica as being about as good as ordinary survival" (Parfit 1986, 201).

My intuitions about this case are very different. The news of *my* impending death on Earth would be devastating. I don't think I would find consolation in talking with my replica. In fact, I am not sure I would like the idea of his loving my wife and taking care of my children. Would my family even care or grieve that I had gone? I don't think I would have much concern for my replica, because it would be *me* that would be dying. As in McMahan's Suicide Case, there would be no question that, if I could switch places with my replica and have him die in a few days instead of me, I would do so in a flash.

What are we to make of these very different intuitions about the hypothetical cases? Presumably, they reflect some deeper views about our understanding of persons and personal identity. If the intuitions are sound, then presumably we should be able to explain what makes them sound by appealing to other arguments and theoretical considerations. Indeed, this is what Parfit, Unger, and others have done. We therefore need to examine these other arguments and the more theoretical considerations offered to support them to decide which intuitions may have better support. It may turn out, of course, that we cannot clearly determine this, in part because we cannot clearly determine which one of various competing theories is best.

It is beyond the scope of this work to offer a comprehensive analysis of these alternative views. The focus of this chapter is on the qualitative view of persons that finds its contemporary expression most clearly in Parfit's work and on pushing the evaluative project a step further. Besides pointing to the conflicting intuitions about the thought experiments, I propose additional reasons for rejecting Parfit's qualitative view of persons and therewith the view that underlies the biological paradigm of death, focusing on what I think are two of the more serious difficulties for Parfit's view. The constitutive view of person is not beset by those same difficulties and is therefore a preferable alternative.

Parfit's view is, at bottom, a contemporary development of Locke's (and Hume's) ideas on personal identity, so it should be no surprise that the criticisms made against Locke's account would find contemporary expression directed against Parfit. I begin with Bishop Joseph Butler's charge of circularity in Locke's view—namely, that any theory of personal identity that relies on memory or psychological continuity must already presuppose an account of personal identity. Parfit's strategy for dealing with this objection, by his reliance on the concept of quasi-memory and his attempt to give a purely causal account of psychological continuity without reference to persons, fails.

There is a related problem for Parfit's attempt to reduce personal identity to psychological continuity: we cannot identify and describe mental states without referring to the person who has them, and the unity of a mental life cannot be explained in an impersonal way. These issues are discussed by Christine Korsgaard and Simon Blackburn, and they lead to broader considerations of how metaphysics and moral philosophy must interrelate in the formulation of a theory about persons and personal identity.[11]

The second difficulty for Parfit's view, after the problem of circularity, concerns the notion of "qualitative similarity" underlying his claim that all that really matters to us about personal identity would be preserved by psychological continuity with any cause. Parfit understands qualitative similarity as a kind of similarity of properties that would be achieved by replication. Just as a photocopy machine may make qualitatively identical copies of a document, the teletransporter may make qualitatively identical copies of a person. Parfit then claims that such qualitative similarity of our psychological states would be all that matters to us about our identity. This assumes, however, that there are no essential, relational properties of persons that might not be preserved by replication. For, if persons have essential relational properties, then even though an original and replica may be qualitatively similar in many internal or nonrelational respects, they may not be qualitatively similar in their relational respects. For example, a forged twenty-dollar bill may be qualitatively similar in many respects to a real twenty-dollar bill, but all that matters to us about the real twenty-dollar bill would not be preserved by replicating it. Persons, like twenty-dollar bills, have essential relational properties insofar as they are essentially social and cultural beings. Moreover, the instantiation of these properties depends on conventions, moral and legal theory, and other aspects of culture (Lizza 1991; Harré 1984; Baker 2000). In other words, persons and their identity are in part defined by the moral and cultural context in which they appear. The conclusions that Parfit draws from the thought experiments are faulty because he ignores this relational dimension of persons.

THE PROBLEM OF CIRCULARITY

Bishop Butler ([1736] 1975) agreed with Locke that memory is a natural way in which we "ascertain our personal identity to ourselves." Butler argued, however, that memory cannot make or constitute personal identity, since our understanding of memory presupposes that there is something else in which personal identity consists. For something to be a memory, it must be the case that the person who remembers something has actually experienced what she claims to remember. If the person did not have the experience that she claims to remember, then it would not make sense to say that the person remembered the event. There must be something else, other than memory, that determines the identity of the person over time. In other words, if I remember winning a race in the third grade, then this presupposes I won the race in the third grade. If I didn't actually win the race, then it cannot be said that I remember winning the race. Thus, my identity with the person who won the race is presupposed and determines whether I have a memory of winning the race. In Butler's words, "One should really think it self-evident, that consciousness of personal identity presupposes, and therefore cannot constitute, personal identity, any more than knowledge, in any other case, can constitute truth, which it presupposes" (Butler [1736] 1975, 100).

If personal identity is actually presupposed by memory, then the possibility of reducing personal identity to forms of psychological continuity, including memories, seems doomed. Parfit has tried to respond to this circularity objection by invoking the notion of "q-memory" or "quasi-memory." He defines "q-memory" as follows: "I am q-remembering an experience if (1) I have a belief about a past experience which seems in itself like a memory belief, (2) someone did have such an experience, and (3) my belief is dependent upon this experience in the same way (whatever that is) in which a memory of an experience is dependent on it" (Parfit [1971] 1975, 209). Q-memory leaves open the possibility that the person who q-remembers an event might not be the same person as the person who experienced the event. Thus, q-memory does not presuppose personal identity. Since every memory is a q-memory, Parfit proposes that we "drop the concept of memory and use in its place the wider concept q-memory." If we did this, "we should describe the relation between an experience and what we now call a 'memory' of this experience in a way which does not presuppose that they are had by the same person" (210). By substituting q-memory for memory, Parfit hopes to introduce a noncircular causal account of personal identity. If a present experience is appropriately caused by a past experience, where this notion of causal connection does not rely on some independent notion of personal identity, then these experiences are experiences of the same person. In fact, according to Parfit, persons are not anything over and above a set or Humean "bundle" of experiences with the appropriate causal relations.

The main difficulty for this approach is whether condition (3) can be coherently spelled out without presupposing some other account of personal identity. For example, suppose I won the race in the third grade but have totally forgotten about it. Years later, my brother reminds me about my winning the race; however, I soon forget his telling me this. Years later, I seem to remember winning the race. But my seeming to remember is caused by my brother's having told me about it and not by my experience of having won the race. Is my seeming to remember winning the race a q-memory? Conditions (1) and (2) seem to be satisfied, but it is unclear whether condition (3) is satisfied, since my seeming to remember was caused not by my experience of winning the race but by my brother's reminding me of it. To distinguish this apparent q-memory from a genuine q-memory—that is, to articulate the right way in which a q-memory is dependent on an experience—we are forced to appeal to whether the causal route leading to my seeming to remember passed through my brother or me. The problem is that, in relying on the distinction between my brother and me, we presuppose a notion of personal identity that we were trying to account for by the causal relations in q-memories. Thus, in determining whether someone has a q-memory, we seem to have to rely on or presuppose an independent notion of personal identity. Butler's criticism resurfaces.

Colin McGinn has pointed out the same difficulty for Parfit's causal account of personal identity: "Since it is perfectly possible for there to be relations of causal dependence between mental states of distinct persons—as when one person comes to have a belief as a result of what another says—we clearly need some restrictions on which causal relations are such as to link states of the same person. And it is surprisingly difficult to supply any restrictions which do not import circularity and yet have a chance of working" (McGinn 1992, 112). Again, the causal account seems insufficient to explain what makes experiences the experiences of the same person.[12]

There is a related difficulty for Parfit's account, namely, P. F. Strawson's argument (1959, 41ff.), suggested by Kant ([1781/1787] 1997, A99–106), that we cannot identify and describe mental states without referring to the person who has them and that the unity of a mental life cannot be explained in an impersonal way. Simon Blackburn nicely summarizes Kant's argument:

> We concentrate on the fundamental capacity of conceiving of experience as experience of a world of independently spatially arrayed objects. This is not possible without organization or synthesis, and Kant distinguishes three stages: the synthesis of apprehension, which is just the emergence of appearances in consciousness; synthesis in imagination, or memory, which is the building up of the enduring three-dimensional object from the successive perceptions of its parts; and finally synthesis of recognition in a concept, which is the recognition of numerical identity of perceived object in the succession of experiences. The aim is to show that such synthesis is at the same time the synthesis of self-consciousness: the feat of seeing experience as experience of a spatially arranged objective world is at the same time the feat of seeing myself as one entity within that world, with a distinctive spatial position and history in time. Without that self-consciousness, the succession of experiences would remain unconceptualized: it is this synthesis that alone prevents experience from being a "rhapsody of perceptions" . . .
>
> The argument now proceeds to another stage . . . Furthermore, it is essential to our mastery of the concepts of space and time that we can make them [certain discriminations]. The ability is to distinguish between similar scenes at different places, and to use the fact of our own location to determine whether a memory was of one or another thing at a time. If we did not do this, we could not give a determinate content to memory as memory of a particular thing, since there would be no anchorage of the original experience to one object or another. This anchorage is given by a unified self subject to a speed limit in space, whose position at different times determines possible objects of memory. (Blackburn 1987, 187–88)

Blackburn thinks, however that the Strawson/Kant argument is not inimical to Parfit:

> The general drift is not towards giving myself a foundational unity through time, but towards seeing awareness of my point of view as one position in space, identified, like all positions, by the stable spatial relations of objects. My experience is indeed experienced from a point of view; this point of view is itself located, as are the objects it presents, and like them—in fact exactly like the one I think of as my body—it moves only in restricted regions at restricted speeds. But no special unity of the subject emerges from these thoughts, because nothing is needed by way of unity or identity or speed limit of the subject beyond what is also needed by way of stability in other objects in space. And for this nothing is required beyond the stability of my body. But we are familiar with the thought that the identity through time of my body is not an all-or-nothing matter, that it will permit of borderlines and slippery slope arguments, and in some actual or imagined circumstances there will be no unique right answer as to whether it has survived or not. We cannot judge the hard-edged quality of the unity reaction this way . . . any appearance of a need for irreducible reference to a self in our thought is in fact superficial, explicable through the need for nothing more than a stable location or point of view, conceived of as that from which the information about the world is gathered. (188–89)

Blackburn's defense of Parfit, however, begs the question. While a body is necessary for a point of view, it may not be sufficient for understanding what it is to have a point of view (Nagel 1979; McTaggart 1927) and what makes a point of view necessarily *my* point of view and no one else's. As noted in chapter 4, Strawson ([1958] 1991) rejects the possibility that we can understand what it means for all experiences to be had by a certain person by referring to a certain body on which the experiences are contingently dependent. For then it could not be consistently maintained that "all the experiences of person P" means the same thing as "all experiences contingently dependent on a certain body B." This latter proposition about the meaning of the experiences of a person (what makes a group of experiences *my* experiences) would then be analytic and not contingent as originally intended. The theorist intends to refer to a group of experiences that are contingently dependent on a certain body. But in order to refer to those experiences, the theorist must assume that what defines the group of experiences is that they are the experiences *of* some person and no one else's. Thus, in order to state the claim that a certain body could explain what it means for my experiences to be my experiences, one must have already identified the experiences as belonging to some person. The theory thus presupposes what it intends to deny—that is, persons in the sense of subjects who nontransferably own their experiences.

Blackburn goes on to point out that, in positing the transcendental ego as what accompanies and gives unity to all apperceptions and as something prior to empirical consciousness, Kant's concern was to emphasize the place of agency in thought. Blackburn states, "the unity of consciousness with which he [Kant] is concerned is the unity of an act bringing into being any determinate combination of the manifold. But action here is not contrasted with cognition. Without action no understanding, and hence no judgement or experience, is possible" (Blackburn 1987, 190). Blackburn does not find this line of thought promising, as he thinks it leads to "a hopelessly transcendental self: a thing whose judging operations are responsible for time itself, and whose noumenal freedom is incompatible with the sway of determinism over the entire world that we know" (191). He thinks that, if Kant is right that agency and judgment are incompatible with a Humean/Parfitian ontology, then we should accept the Humean/Parfitian ontology and downgrade this strand in Kant to, at best, a necessary illusion required for thinking of ourselves as other than passive.

Christine Korsgaard also discusses whether Parfit's view conflicts with the notion of agency that Kant presupposed as necessary to making sense of free choice and moral responsibility. Her conclusions differ from Blackburn's. According to Korsgaard (1989), Kant thought that, as rational beings, we can view ourselves from two standpoints: (1) as natural phenomena whose behavior may be causally explained and predicted and (2) as agents who think and originate actions:

> These two standpoints cannot be completely assimilated to each other, and the way we view ourselves when we occupy one can appear incongruous with the way we view ourselves when we occupy the other. As objects of theoretical study, we see ourselves as wholly determined by natural forces, the mere undergoers of our experiences. Yet as agents, we view ourselves as free and responsible, as authors of our actions and the *leaders* of our lives. The incongruity need not become contradiction. So long as we keep in mind that the two different views of ourselves spring from two different relations in which we stand to our actions . . . These two relations to our actions are equally legitimate, inescapable, and governed by reason, but they are separate. Kant does not assert that it is a matter of theoretical fact that we are agents, that we are free, and that we are responsible. Rather, we must view ourselves in this way when we occupy the standpoint of practical reason — that is, when we are deciding what to do. This follows from the fact that we must regard ourselves as the causes — the first cause — of the things that we will. And this fundamental attitude is forced upon us by the necessity of making choices, regardless of the theoretical or metaphysical facts. (120)

This leads Korsgaard to a criticism of Parfit's view of personal identity:

> From the theoretical standpoint, an action may be viewed as just another experience, and the assertion that it has a subject may be, as Parfit says, "because of the way we talk." But from the practical point of view, actions and choices must be viewed as having agents and choosers. This is what *makes* them, in our eyes, our own actions and choices rather than events that befall us. In fact, it is only from the practical point of view that actions and choices can be distinguished from mere "behavior" determined by biological and psychological laws. This does not mean that our existence as agents is asserted as a further fact or requires a separately existing entity that should be discernible from the theoretical point of view. It is rather that from the practical point of view our relationship to our actions and choices is essentially *authorial*: from it, we view them as *our own*. I believe that when we think about the way in which our own lives matter to us personally, we think of ourselves in this way. We think of living our lives, and even of having our experiences, as something that we *do*. And it is this important feature of our sense of our identity that Parfit's account leaves out. (120–21)

Korsgaard has tried to separate the ontological question, such as whether persons are "deeply or metaphysically separated" in a Cartesian sense or reducible to psychological continuity without reference to persons, from the practical question of whether we need to think of ourselves as agents and free choosers in order to act. However, her separation of the ontological and ethical issues is untenable. I agree with Blackburn that there is a conflict. If Korsgaard allows Parfit's claim that talk about a subject of experience is just talk, then it would seem that Parfit could equally respond that talk about an authorial relation to our actions or regarding ourselves as the first cause of what we will may also be just talk. Korsgaard is right that Kant did not claim to know that we are free, responsible agents, but he also claimed that he did not know whether a single human action was ever morally good (Kant [1785] 1993). The ontological and ethical claims are mutually dependent. A world in which there is talk of but no real freedom is a world in which there is talk of but no real morality. If we think we should accept a theory of morality that includes postulating autonomous agents or transcendental egos, then we should accept an ontology that postulates subjects (persons) that is compatible with this moral theory. It is hard to see how the Humean/Parfitian reductionist ontology is compatible with such a theory, since it views persons only from the standpoint of beings whose nature and behavior can be wholly explained and predicted in nonsubjective, naturalistic terms. Positing a non-eliminable subject of experience whose identity is not a matter of degree and who can act freely may be necessary for moral explanation. This may not necessarily entail accepting Cartesian egos. But it does seem to entail accepting the idea that persons, human agency, and morality cannot be understood entirely in the third-person terms of the sciences of physics and biology. It seems to entail accepting a nonreductive view of persons.

QUALITATIVE SIMILARITY AND
PSYCHOLOGICAL CONTINUITY

Immediately after presenting his case involving teletransportation, Parfit distinguishes qualitative from numerical identity: "There are two kinds of sameness. I and my Replica are qualitatively identical, or exactly alike. But we may not be numerically identical, or one and the same person. Similarly, two white billiard balls are not numerically identical but may be qualitatively identical. If I paint one of these balls red, it will not now be qualitatively identical to itself yesterday. But the red ball that I see now and the white ball that I painted red are numerically identical. They are one and the same ball" (Parfit 1986, 201).

Having assumed that he and his replica would be qualitatively identical, Parfit describes versions of the two traditional criteria of personal identity: physical continuity and psychological continuity. He then discusses how teletransportation could be evaluated by using the psychological criterion. According to Parfit, the physical criterion states:

> (1) What is necessary is not the continued existence of the whole body, but the continued existence of enough of the brain to be the brain of a living person. X today is one and the same person as Y at some past time if and only if (2) enough of Y's brain continued to exist, and is now X's brain, and (3) there does not exist a different person who also has enough of Y's brain. (4) Personal identity over time just consists in the holding of facts like (2) and (3). (Parfit 1986, 204)

The psychological criterion states:

> (1) there is psychological continuity if and only if there are overlapping chains of strong connectedness. X today is one and the same person as Y at some past time if and only if (2) X is psychologically continuous with Y, (3) this continuity has the right kind of cause and (4) there does not yet exist a different person who is also psychologically continuous with Y. Personal identity over time just consists in the holding of facts like (2) to (4). (207)

Parfit asserts that there are three versions of the psychological criterion, which differ in the question of "the right kind of cause" mentioned in condition (3). "On the Narrow version," he writes, "this must be the normal cause. On the Wide version, this could be any reliable cause. On the Widest version, the cause could be any cause" (207). On the narrow version, the normal cause of psychological continuity involves the continued existence of the brain. Brain continuity is thus a necessary but not sufficient condition for personal identity. On the two wide versions, the cause need not involve the continued existence of the brain. Thus, reconsidering his imaginary story in which his brain and body are destroyed, Parfit writes, "The Scanner and the Replicator produce a person who has a new but exactly similar brain and body, and who is psychologically continuous with me as I was when I pressed the green button. The cause of this continuity is, though unusual, reliable. On both the Physical Criterion and the Narrow Psychological Criterion, my Replica would not be me. On the two Wide Criteria, he would be me" (208).

Parfit assumes that all of a person's psychological features depend on the states of the cells in the person's brain and nervous system and that an organic replica of him would be psychologically exactly like him. He thinks we need not decide between the three versions of the psychological criterion, since any difference between his brain and that of his replica would not give rise to a significant difference in their psychological states. He concludes that we can therefore accept even the widest version of the psychological criterion. If we consider the branch-line case, in which Parfit remains on Earth and his replica exists on Mars, Parfit believes the psychological continuity between him at t_1 on Earth and his replica at t_2 on Mars is "just as good as" the psychological continuity between him at t_1 on Earth and him at t_2 on Earth.

Parfit's account, however, fails to take into consideration the essential relational qualities of persons, which may differ for the replica on Mars and the original on Earth, even if many or all of their intrinsic or nonrelational qualities are exactly similar. Earlier, I offered by analogy the example of the difference between bona fide, U.S.-minted twenty-dollar bills and illicit exact duplicates. What matters about twenty-dollar bills is not simply qualitative similarity. Currency has essential, relational properties. It cannot exist except in relation to an economic and political system. Its causal history and how it functions in a network of economic exchange is essential to its being the kind of thing that it is. Forged twenty-dollar bills, no matter how similar their internal properties to genuine bills, are not currency. To be genuine bills, they must be recognized as such within the economic system. The causal history of the forged bills precludes this recognition.

So it is with persons. Because we are essentially moral, social, and cultural beings, our identity is in part determined by the relations we have to others. Personal identity or survival is not purely an internal matter of bodily or psychological continuity. Moreover, whether personal identity is all-or-nothing or a matter of degree may depend on moral, social, and cultural considerations.[13]

It takes only a little imagination to envision problematic cases in an age of replication in which we would think identity, not survival, would matter. These cases suggest that we would not give up a determinate concept of personal identity in favor of survival. Imagine armies of replicas of Derek Parfit. What would we have to say about them? How, for example, would inheritance laws apply to them? What legal and moral status would they have? Would a replica of Derek Parfit be morally and legally responsible for the actions of the original Derek Parfit? Would parental and spousal obligations carry over to replicas, and if so, to one, some, or all of them? Suppose one replica were defective in some way. Would it be morally and legally acceptable to terminate its life as long as the other replicas remained alive? What rights, if any, would we accord replicas? Would they be "human rights"?[14]

Our inability to readily answer these important questions points to what is essentially flawed in trying to conclude anything about persons from consideration of some of Parfit's thought experiments. We are asked for our intuition about these hypothetical cases without any moral, social, and cultural context in which to judge them. We have no idea of what the context would be in an age of replication, so we cannot give meaningful responses to the hypothetical scenarios. The value of a crucial variable is missing. Would society regard and treat replicas as persons? Or, for whatever reasons, would it regard and treat replicas in much the same way it currently treats replicas (i.e., forgeries) of twenty-dollar bills?

When Parfit asks whether I would consider my replica on Mars to be me and to be continuing my life, I may wish it to be true because the only alternative is my death. If I also consider how society might treat replicas and appreciate the rationale behind such treatment, my view might change. For example, if society outlawed replication and treated replicas as organic forgeries, I might believe my replica would neither be a person nor continue my life. In the branch-line case, such laws would reinforce my conviction that my survival and identity have little to do with my replica on Mars. Similarly, consider the reactions to forged twenty-dollar bills from different perspectives. The counterfeiter certainly wishes the forgeries to pass as genuine bills. Internal, nonrelational qualitative similarity and personal economic benefit are "what matter" to the counterfeiter. The secretary of the treasury, however, has different concerns; qualitative similarity is not enough.

A more fundamental point that grounds this challenge to the thought experiments is the thesis that facts external to the person are essential to identifying the content of a person's mental states, such as beliefs, desires, attitudes, aims, and projects (Burge [1979] 1991, 1988). If the identity conditions of these mental states are dependent on conditions external to the person's subjective awareness of them, then we would need to know about the external conditions to decide questions about psychological continuity and personal identity over time.

Suppose your relationship to your family is very important to your subjective sense of who you are. Suppose further that certain projects are very important to you, that you "identify" yourself with certain political and social causes. Now consider the branch-line case. You are told that your replica on Mars will be treated in a way that is radically different from the way you are currently treated. For example, your replica will not be allowed to see your family and will be restricted from participating in the causes with which you so passionately identify. Because of certain cultural conventions in the age of replication, the replica's attitudes and projects become entirely unrealistic and impractical.

In contrast, the attitudes, aims, and projects of the entity that continues to exist on Earth will remain as realistic and practical as they were before you stepped into the New Scanner. It seems clear that, if you subjectively identified yourself with certain realistic attitudes, aims, and projects, then you would have a rational basis for identifying yourself with the entity on Earth rather than on Mars. In fact, you would have reason for denying your psychological continuity with the replica on Mars, since that entity, no matter how insistently it may claim to have the same realistic attitudes, plans, and projects that you had before entering the Scanner, simply does not have those same realistic attitudes, aims, and projects. External factors have made what the replica subjectively identifies as its attitudes, aims, and projects completely unrealistic. Moreover, the replica would soon realize this fact and likely abandon those attitudes, plans, and projects for new ones. Its subjective sense of itself would change.

In short, even if psychological continuity is what matters to us about our identity, it may be destroyed in the process of replication, not because replication fails to preserve the nonrelational, qualitative similarity of our psychological states but because those states are essentially relational: they are dependent on circumstances external to the person. In fact, it is hard to imagine how the replica's, say, central concern for a family would be qualitatively the same as that of the original person, especially if the replica were aware that it could not relate to family members in the way the original related to them. The replica would not "feel" the closeness of its family in the same way the original does. As we multiply this kind of change for a range of psychological states of the original, we have more and more reason for thinking that psychological continuity would not be preserved by replication.

Finally, suggesting that there would be no problem if we considered only the nonbranching form of replication will not do. Replication of persons, in principle, threatens our moral, legal, and cultural systems of thought in such a fundamental way that our concept of person might require such radical modification that it would no longer be the same concept. For this reason, I find the thought experiments involving replication meaningless. Since we have no idea what the moral, legal, and cultural context would be in an age of replication, we cannot evaluate our current intuitions about the hypothetical cases involving replication. The background conditions that give meaning to the concept of person are so unspecified that the thought experiments are useless.

This same problem infects, to some degree, thought experiments in which we consider the possibility of replacement of our brains with exact duplicates. "Suppose," Parfit asks, "that I need surgery. All of my cells have a defect which, in time, would be fatal. But a surgeon can replace all these cells. He can insert new cells that are exact replicas of the existing cells except that they have no defect" (Parfit 1986, 474). Parfit then proposes two ways in which the surgery might be done, to challenge the importance of physical continuity to personal identity. In both cases, he assumes that psychological continuity would be preserved: "In *Case One*, the surgeon performs a hundred operations. In each of these, he removes a hundredth part of my brain, and inserts a replica of this part. In *Case Two*, the surgeon follows a different procedure. He first removes all of the parts of my brain, and then inserts all of their replicas" (474). As Jeff McMahan points out, "Parfit concedes that his brain would survive in Case One but not in Case Two. But he argues that the difference between the two cases can be seen, upon reflection, to be trivial. 'The difference between the cases,' he writes, 'is merely . . . a difference in the ordering and the removals and insertions. In Case One, the surgeon alternates between removing and inserting. In Case Two, he does all the removing before the inserting. Can *this*,' he asks, 'be the difference between life and death? . . . Can it be so important, for my survival, whether the new parts are, for a time, joined to the old parts?'" (McMahan 2002, 70).

Parfit's intuition is that he would survive the surgery in both cases, since his psychological continuity would be preserved. He therefore concludes that physical brain continuity is not necessary for personal identity. McMahan's intuitions are different. He believes that, just as one would not have egoistic concern for a replica of oneself, there would be no basis for egoistic concern about a person who had a replica of one's entire brain as in Case Two. Case Two is as bad as ordinary death. However, in Case One, McMahan thinks egoistic concern for oneself tomorrow would not be compromised by the loss of one-hundredth of one's brain today, provided the rest of the brain continued to support consciousness and mental activity.

McMahan is not sure what to make of this intuitive disagreement. He thinks Parfit described the difference in the two cases in a way that suggests the difference could not be important. McMahan thinks it is unclear which view is more reasonable and suggests that both views are within the range of plausibility.

I want to suggest that there is more to the matter: attention needs to be paid to the background conditions under which the hypothetical is presented and to the relational qualities of persons. I think McMahan's intuition that personal identity would be preserved in Case One but not in Case Two can be supported on the basis of nontrivial reasons if we pay attention to these background factors. If we assume that many of our normal social, legal, and cultural relations assume uniqueness of persons and would be threatened by the possibility of replicas (analogous to the way our economic system would be threatened by forged currency), there seems to be good reason to deny that whatever gets preserved by replication of our brains and psychological continuity is *all* that matters in terms of personal identity. We can imagine laws that would be designed to ensure uniqueness of persons and would invoke criteria, such as sameness of brain or body, to ensure that uniqueness. The "trivial" difference in how the operations take place might not be trivial at all, given the aims and rationale for a rule that distinguishes the two cases in order to preserve uniqueness.

Parfit tries to support his view by analogizing the issue raised about persons in the brain replacement cases to the existence of a club:

> Consider a club that is limited to fifty members. All of the existing members want to resign. Fifty other people want to join this club. There is a rule that a new member cannot be admitted unless in the presence of forty-nine existing members. Because of this rule, the club continues to exist only if what happens is like Case One. What happens must be this. One member resigns and a new member is admitted. Another member resigns and a new member is admitted. A third member resigns and a new member is admitted. At the end of this series, this club would still exist, with entirely new members. Suppose instead that what happens is like Case Two. All of the old members resign. Because of the rule, the new members cannot now be admitted. The club ceases to exist. (Parfit 1986, 495)

The implication of the example is that, just as it seems silly to say that the club exists if the members are replaced gradually but not if they are replaced all at once, it is silly to think that whether the person continues to exist depends on how the brain cells are replaced. Parfit concludes his discussion with the following *reductio ad absurdum* argument:

> Can *this* difference be the difference between life and death? Can *my* fate depend on this difference between the ordering of the removals and insertions? Can it be so important for my survival, whether the new parts are, for a time, joined to the old parts? This could make all the difference if it produced some further fact. This would be so

if my survival was like some sacred power, which one priest could give to another only by ritual involving touch. But there is no such further fact. There is merely the fact that, if the new parts are for a time joined to the old parts, we describe the resulting brain as the same brain. If the new parts are not so joined, we describe the resulting brain as a different brain. (495)

One way to respond to a *reductio ad absurdum* argument is to embrace the conclusion and show that it is not as implausible as it seems. This is the strategy I wish to take here. A better example than the priest's touch as the mark between life and death might be the Hindu son's breaking the skull of the cremated parent to release the soul from the body (Kalitzkus 2004, 144). My point is that Parfit's hypothetical cases ignore the moral, legal, and cultural values and the background conditions that are relevant to evaluating the cases. The significance of the Hindu son's breaking of the skull needs to be interpreted in the light of the Hindu belief system and values. It is too quick to conclude that the son's action is trivial and cannot be what distinguishes life from death. The son's action might derive moral and ontological significance in the light of other beliefs and values. Assuming that all that matters to Hindus about persons is psychological continuity begs the question.

Similarly, we can ask why the club would have such a rule for change of membership. As presented, it sounds like a stupid rule, but it may not be a stupid rule at all. For example, suppose financial interests were at stake in maintaining the club at fifty members for an extended period of time. There happen to be fifty people ready and willing to join the club at a certain time, but this is extraordinarily unusual. Normally, the club has difficulty finding new members so the club has devised the rule to ensure that the membership will remain constant. Or perhaps the rule was imposed on the club as a condition of its formation by some other group that had a contractual, financial relationship with the club. Given these conditions and the interests and values at stake, relational facts about the club are relevant to its conditions of identity. In this context, it would not be silly to say that the club continued to exist if the membership were replaced gradually but not if all at once.

THE COMBINED SPECTRUM

A similar difficulty plagues the thought experiment involving the Combined Spectrum, which Parfit uses to support his claim that personal identity may be indeterminate or a matter of degree. This thought experiment fails because relevant moral and cultural conditions are radically unspecified. Any respectable intuitions about this case, I believe, are dependent on consideration of moral and cultural factors. This criticism of the thought experiment, in turn, shows that our identity is in part determined by such factors. Consideration of our current moral, legal, and cultural beliefs supports the idea that our identity must be determinate and that identity, rather than survival, is what matters.

The Combined Spectrum involves all of the possible variations in the degrees of both physical and psychological connectedness:

> At the near end of this spectrum is the normal case in which a future person would be fully continuous with me as I am now, both physically and psychologically. This person would be me in just the way that, in my actual life, it will be me who wakes up tomorrow. At the far end of this spectrum the resulting person would have no continuity with me as I am now, either physically or psychologically. In this case the scientists would destroy my brain and body, and then create, out of new organic matter, a perfect Replica of someone else. We can suppose that, when Garbo was 30, a group of scientists recorded the states of all the cells in her brain and body.
>
> In the first case in this spectrum, at the near end, nothing would be done. In the second case, a few of the cells in my brain and body would be replaced. The new cells would *not* be exact duplicates. As a result, there would be somewhat less psychological connectedness between me and the person who wakes up. This person would not have all of my memories, and his character would in one way be unlike mine. He would have some apparent memories of Greta Garbo's life, and have one of Garbo's characteristics. Unlike me he would enjoy acting. His body would also be in one way less like mine, and more like Garbo's. His eyes would be more like Garbo's eyes. Further along the spectrum, a larger percentage of my cells would be replaced with dissimilar cells. The resulting person would be in fewer ways psychologically connected with me, and in more ways connected with Garbo, as she was at the age of 30. And there would be similar changes in this person's body. Near the far end, most of my cells would be replaced with dissimilar cells. The person who wakes up would have only a few of the cells in my original brain and body, and between her and me there would be only a few psychological connections. She would have a few apparent memories that fit my past, and a few of my habits and desires. But in every other way she would be, both physically and psychologically, just like Greta Garbo. (Parfit 1986, 236–37)

Parfit claims there are three possible responses to the Combined Spectrum case. (1) We can adopt the reductionist view and hold that the question of whether one continues to exist over the range of the spectrum does not have an answer (i.e., it is an empty question). (2) We can believe there is a sharp borderline between being me and being someone else, even though in some cases we may not know where that borderline is. Or (3) we can believe that, in all cases in the spectrum, the resulting person would be me.

For Parfit, the third response is the least plausible, because at the far end of the spectrum there is absolutely no physical or psychological connection between Parfit at t_1 and Garbo at some later time. In this case, the scientist destroys Parfit's brain and body and makes Garbo out of completely new matter.

Parfit also argues against response (2), since he believes there is no significant, nontrivial borderline on the spectrum at which we would be justified in saying that Parfit ceased to be Parfit and became Garbo. According to Parfit, if we chose (2) we would be forced to accept the following claims:

> Somewhere in this Spectrum, there is a sharp borderline. There must be some critical set of the cells replaced, and some critical degree of psychological change, which would make all the difference. If the surgeons replace slightly fewer than these cells, and produce one fewer psychological change, it will be me who wakes up. If they replace the few extra cells, and produce one more psychological change, I shall cease to exist, and the person waking up would be someone else. There must be such a pair of cases somewhere in this spectrum, *even though there could never be any evidence where these cases are.* (238–39)

These claims are very hard to believe, Parfit asserts, since it is hard to believe the difference between life and death would consist in the very small differences he describes. According to Parfit, we believe there must be a *deep* difference between some future person's being me and his being someone else; but the differences between any two neighboring cases in this Spectrum are trivial. Parfit concludes that (1), the reductionist response, is therefore the most plausible. In this view, it would be an empty question whether the resulting person in the central cases in the Combined Spectrum would be Parfit.

Parfit is right in identifying (3) as the least plausible response, but he does not provide a good reason for rejecting (2). Even if one's decision on the borderline cases relied on a "trivial" physical difference, this would not make the decision itself trivial. Arbitrarily picking some point on the Combined Spectrum might derive moral and rational significance from the fact that a point had to be picked, given a background of moral aims and purposes. One might think there must always be a determinate answer to the question of whether a person exists or continues to exist, not for the reason that Cartesian selves exist but for the reason that a moral community could not function without having determinate answers to these questions. In fact, our current moral practice seems to presuppose that personal identity must always be determinate and that identity, not survival, is what matters.

If we were faced with the case of the Combined Spectrum or other hypothetical scenarios such as those involving replication, one of two things would occur: either (1) our current moral practices would have to be radically revised, and the concept of person underlying those practices would accordingly undergo revision, or (2) we would retain our current concept of person as a determinate entity and stipulate conditions for its persistence. In either case, it is difficult to see how we can learn anything about our current concept of person from consideration of Parfit's hypothetical scenarios. With option (1), we would have a very different concept of person, not because of some insight into why our current concept was mistaken but because of changes in moral and legal practices. With option (2), we would believe the difference between life and death consists of very small differences in physiology, similar to the very small difference we find between neighboring cases in the Combined Spectrum or between originals and replicas. There is nothing inconsistent, however, with thinking that this small difference may constitute a very *deep* difference, namely, the difference between the life and death of a person.

Parfit considers option (2) but claims that, if we hold such a view,

> we do not believe that the true criterion of personal identity must draw some sharp borderline somewhere in the Combined Spectrum. Rather we believe that, to avoid incoherence, we should draw such a line.
>
> This view hardly differs from the Reductionist view. If we do draw such a line we cannot believe that it has, intrinsically, either rational or moral significance. We must pick some point on this Spectrum, up to which we will call the resulting person me, and beyond which we will call him someone else. Our choice of this point will have to be arbitrary. We must draw this line between two neighboring cases, though the difference between them is, in itself, trivial. If this is what we do, this should not affect our attitude towards these two cases. It would clearly be irrational for me to regard the first case as being as good as ordinary survival, while regarding the second case as being as bad as ordinary death. When I consider this range of cases, I naturally ask, "Will the resulting person be me?" By drawing our line, we have chosen to *give* an answer to this question. But, since our choice was arbitrary, it cannot justify any claim about what matters. If this is how we answer the question about my identity, we have made it true that, in this range of cases, personal identity is *not* what matters. And this is the most important claim in the Reductionist View. Our view differs only trivially from this view. Reductionists claim that, in some cases, questions about personal identity are indeterminate. We add the claim that, in such cases, we ought to give these questions answers, even if we have to do so in a way that is arbitrary, and that deprives our answers of any significance. I regard this view as one version of Reductionism, the tidy-minded version

that abolishes indeterminacy with uninteresting stipulative definitions. Since the difference is so slight, I shall ignore this version of this view. (241–42)

I disagree. If we think there must or ought to be answers to the questions of personal identity, even if the means of determining those answers may in some cases be arbitrary, then we believe personal identity *is* what matters. It matters for the same reasons that we think we must answer the questions, and these reasons are not trivial. In fact, Parfit himself states that we may be inclined to draw a line along the spectrum "to avoid incoherence." Avoidance of incoherence is not a trivial concern. But what is this "incoherence"? Superficially, it is the incompatibility of believing (1) that questions about personal identity must always be determinate and that personal identity is what matters and (2) that there are no determinate answers to the questions about personal identity raised in certain hypothetical cases and that, therefore, survival is all that matters. On a deeper level, the "incoherence" is the incompatibility of (2) with the reason for believing (1). The reason for believing (1) is that it is presupposed by some of our basic moral concepts and practices. If (2) were true and the hypothetical scenarios occurred, these concepts and practices would be inapplicable. Unless we are willing to abandon these moral concepts and practices in the hypothetical cases and, to be consistent, abandon them in our current practice, we ought not to accept (2). Thus, because there are important reasons for giving determinate answers to the questions of personal identity, it would be *irrational* for us not to regard some point along the Combined Spectrum as being as good as ordinary survival and some later point being as bad as ordinary death.

If the Combined Spectrum is possible, then it is clearly possible that circumstances might arise in which one would need to decide where the borderline lies. Suppose there were some pressing question about whether an individual should be held morally responsible for some action committed before the surgery contemplated in the Combined Spectrum. After the surgery, we need to determine whether that person still exists and should therefore suffer some sanction or punishment. The gravity of the situation requires us to make a decision as to whether we should hold the postoperative person morally responsible. *Someone* must be held accountable, so we arbitrarily stipulate a borderline. Under these circumstances—and given the belief that someone must be held responsible, make restitution, be punished, and so on, in order to maintain public order—such an arbitrary stipulation would be the fair thing to do and therefore the moral and rational thing to do.

We do not have to consider thought experiments to grasp this point. It is evident in actual practice. For example, a similar rationale underlies the U.S. Supreme Court's decision in *Roe v. Wade* (410 U.S. 113 [1973]), which affirms that the state may proscribe abortion after the fetus is viable outside the womb, except when abortion is necessary to preserve the life or health of the mother. In practice, the point of viability is fixed at the end of the second trimester of gestation. Although this point is supposed to coincide with the time when the fetus is viable, the particular point in time is arbitrary in the sense that one could not justify why the selected time was not one day earlier or later by appeal to facts about viability. Within certain parameters of viability, a particular point is picked because a point *has* to be picked, given certain values and aims underlying the decision. Even if viability has some intrinsic value, as some have argued, the particular point at which viability is fixed derives its importance and value from the ethical, social, and political rationale for fixing the point.

In its decision in *Roe v. Wade*, the Court sought to balance the state's interest in the potential life of the fetus and a woman's right to privacy. The Court ruled that the right to privacy was not absolute and that a compelling state interest may limit that right. At issue, then, was at what point the state's interest in protecting the potential life of the fetus becomes "compelling," such that the state would be justified in restricting abortion. The Court ruled that this point was "at viability [which 'is usually placed at about seven months (28 weeks) but may occur earlier, even at 24 weeks']. This is so because the fetus then presumably has the capacity for life outside the mother's womb. State regulation protective of fetal life after viability thus has both logical and biological justifications." The "logical and biological justifications" provide the rationale for fixing viability as the point at which the state's interest in the potential life of the fetus becomes compelling. The rationale for fixing a point in the first place, however, comes from considerations of justice on how to balance legitimate, competing interests.

When it is necessary to balance competing interests, the Court will look for some principled way to draw a line. Some fact, such as "the capacity of meaningful life outside the womb," might be invoked to draw the line. We should bear in mind, however, that this "principled" way to draw the line is justified in part by whether it meets the requirements of justice that mandated drawing the line in the first place. It would be a mistake to imbue *viability* with any kind of value that, in itself, could determine whether the requirements of justice to balance competing interests are met. For example, suppose technology increased to the point where the fetus could be removed and sustained outside the womb several weeks after conception. Would the state then be justified in proscribing abortion at this much earlier point in time? I do not believe so, because a point this early in pregnancy would not allow a woman to exercise her legitimate right to privacy. Thus, viability would not be a "principled" way to fix the point at which the state's interest in protecting potential life became compelling, since this would violate the requirements of justice—that is, a need to fairly balance competing interests—which was what justified drawing a line in the first place. In the interest of justice, some other point would have to be picked. Moreover, even if this point were arbitrary in the sense that it would not have the "biological justification" that the Court claimed for "viability," that alone would not make the point unjustifiable. Its rational justification would come from the fact that, in the interest of justice—a respect for legitimate, competing interests—a point had to be picked.

Now, paraphrasing Parfit, we can ask, should it matter to us whether a fetus happens to fall beyond the "arbitrary" point at which the state's interest in its potential life becomes compelling? Since the choice of the point was arbitrary, Parfit would presumably maintain, as he does in the case of the Combined Spectrum, that "it cannot justify any claim about what matters" and that "it deprives our answers of any significance." If, however, we acknowledge the rationale provided by our theory of justice that justified picking a point, then that same rationale explains why it *should* matter to us whether the fetus falls beyond that point. The fetus's moral, social, and political standing is in part a function of the moral, social, and political context in which it appears. In addition, if one accepts a form of moral realism that holds that the requirements of justice demand picking a point, then it would be an objective, moral fact that the fetus was deserving of protection by the state after that point.

Another example of an actual context in which stipulation of some point derives its moral and rational significance from the fact that a point must be picked is found in the current practice of declaring death on the basis of neurological criteria. Although the letter of the law stipulates that death can be declared on the basis of neurological criteria only when all brain functions have irreversibly ceased, in actual clinical practice death is declared even though some neural activity in the brain may remain (Halevy and Brody 1993; Veatch 1993; Truog 1997). This residual activity is deemed insignificant in terms of indicating the continued life of the person. The drawing of a line of how much neural activity is necessary to indicate life is arbitrary in the sense that one could not appeal to neurological facts to support drawing the line at one point as opposed to a neighboring point. Yet, within the parameters of the definition of death as the cessation of the life of the organism as a whole and acceptance of a neurological criterion for determining death, a point is picked. The decision to draw a line, however, is not arbitrary, but is justified by the aims and values that underlie the acceptance of neurological criteria for determining death.

Before ending this discussion of the Combined Spectrum, I should note that my earlier point about how extrinsic factors can influence whether one would identify oneself with some future person can also be seen in the context of the Combined

Spectrum.[15] Suppose two individuals with different motivations were about to undergo the same, borderline, Garbo-transforming operation. One person, say, Michael, is suicidal and hopes the operation ends his life once and for all. The other, say, myself, hopes to survive the operation and become more like Garbo. We can then ask how our attitudes toward the operation would be affected by some social stipulation about whether we survive the operation.

Suppose part of Michael's reason for committing suicide is to relieve others of the burden of having to care for him. Suppose further that he believes he is worth more dead than alive and that his intention is for his family to collect on his life insurance. He is then told that the law stipulates that he will survive the operation. Thus, his family will still have the burden of caring for him, and his life insurance will not pay off. This stipulation and its consequences should make a difference to Michael about whether he should undergo the operation. Even though the stipulation might be arbitrary, it is significant because his identity and continued existence would be affected by it. If he cannot succeed in his aim of committing suicide through the operation, it would be irrational for him to undergo the operation.

Suppose I am told that the law stipulates that I do not survive the operation and that the postoperative person will be considered to be someone else. Now, suppose part of my motivation for undergoing the operation was to improve my social recognition, especially in terms of how I wish others to remember me after I have died. (Suppose I am one of those people who is more concerned with my legacy than with my current social standing.) I want the Garbo mystique. I want others to regard me and remember me in the way they remember Garbo. Now, because of the legal stipulation, my plan is thwarted. People will think I died during the operation, and I will not be remembered as Garbo-like. In this age of weird operations, the law has ways of dealing with this new mode of generation of individuals. Suppose I learn that the law prohibits the operation, and, if discovered, the postoperative person will be immediately executed. Given these various scenarios, my attitude about whether to undergo the operation will be affected. I will presumably look around for some other way to become more like Garbo. If I identify myself with certain projects, the success of which depends on others, and am told that those projects will be thwarted because of others, then it is reasonable to think my attitude about undertaking those projects will be affected. Whether others regard me as continuing to exist matters to me. My own sense of myself is in part a function of how others regard me.[16]

In sum, psychological continuity does not mean simply the continuity of an internal qualitative similarity of psychological states. Psychological continuity is dependent on facts external to the person's subjective awareness of her psychological states. A person's subjective awareness of her psychological states is contingent on facts about the world in which she lives.

PERSONS AND NATIONS

Parfit sometimes uses the analogy of persons to nations to illustrate his reductionist view about persons.[17] He classifies as reductionists those who accept that

(3)   A person's existence just consists in the existence of a brain and a body, and the occurrence of a series of interrelated physical and mental events,

but who also hold that

(5)   A person is an entity that is distinct from a brain and a body, and such a series of events. (Parfit 1986, 211)

"On this version of the Reductionist View," Parfit writes, "a person is not merely a composite object, with these various components. A person is an entity that has a brain and body, and has particular thoughts, desires, and so on. But, though (5) is true, a person is not a separately existing entity. Though (5) is true, (3) is also true" (211).

An ambiguity may be thought to arise from Parfit's failure to explicate the sense in which such theorists maintain that a person is "not merely a composite object" but "not a separately existing entity." Parfit admits that this version of reductionism seems self-contradictory. He invokes Hume to support his claim that (3) and (5) are consistent:

It may help to consider Hume's analogy: "I cannot compare the soul more properly to anything than to a republic, or commonwealth." Most of us are Reductionists about nations. We would accept the following claims: Nations exist. Ruritania does not exist, but France does. Though nations exist, a nation is not an entity that exists separately, apart from its citizens and its territory. We would accept

(6)   A nation's existence just involves the existence of its citizens, living together in certain ways, on its territory.

Some claim

(7)   A nation just is these citizens and this territory.

Others claim

(8)   A nation is an entity that is distinct from its citizens and its territory. (211–12)

Parfit maintains that we may believe (8) and (6) are consistent and, by analogy, that (3) and (5) are also consistent.

The problem, however, is that we need to know in what sense (8) claims that a nation is an entity distinct from (i.e., nonidentical to) its citizens and territory. If the nation is not identical to its citizens and territory, as (8) states, then what is the relationship between the nation and its citizens and territory? Similarly, if a person is not identical to its brain, body, and a series of interrelated physical and mental events, what is the nature of this relationship? The difference between (7) and (8) is not a mere difference of *façon de parler*. Proposition (7) states that an identity relation holds between the nation and its citizens, whereas (8) suggests something else. Parfit does not explore the nature of this relationship but assumes that it would not be any less reductive than the identity relationship and, consequently, that it could not support the view that persons are entities whose existence must be all-or-nothing. If, as I have maintained, the relationship is that of constitution, then persons and nations may have essential relational properties such that we should deny (6) and by analogy the claim that a person's existence just consists in the existence of a brain and a body and the occurrence of a series of interrelated mental and physical events.

A nation's existence does not just involve the internal relations of its citizens living on some territory. It also involves relationships between those citizens and the citizens of other nations. Consider the following questions. When does a nation, say, Israel, come into existence? Does the existence of Palestinians living together on certain territory suffice for the nation of Palestine to exist? What about the Mohawk nation or Quebec? This is not just a linguistic matter. Various moral, legal, and political arguments could be advanced in support of different answers to these questions. When and whether we consider a group of citizens living on territory to be a nation will therefore depend on which arguments we find persuasive. Moreover, there may be good legal and political reasons to treat the existence of a nation as all-or-nothing rather than as a matter of degree. One reason is given by Korsgaard, when she uses the term *state* rather than *nation* (Korsgaard 1989). *State*, more than *nation*, connotes the idea of agency, and agency presupposes unity and a responsible subject.

Torbjörn Tännsjö challenges Parfit's thought along similar lines by emphasizing the centrality of personal identity in certain moral theories and how those theories treat a person as an all-or-nothing kind of being rather than a being that can exist in degrees. Tännsjö observes that some philosophers, like Parfit, have thought that the answer to the metaphysical question of who we are should rationally influence our moral outlook. Other philosophers, including Kant and Locke (cf. my earlier remarks about Locke's recognition that *person* is a *forensic* term), have thought that the notion of person is fundamentally a moral one and that our moral beliefs ought to determine our beliefs about who and what we are. Thus, as indicated above, Kant thought that, to make sense of moral responsibility and free will, we need to hypothesize a "noumenal" self. Tännsjö sides with Kant and Locke. He believes that "metaphysics and moral philosophy cannot be pursued in isolation from each other," but he states, "Parfit to the contrary notwithstanding, moral considerations ought to determine our view of personal identity and not the other way around."[18]

Tännsjö challenges Parfit's reductionist claim that everything that is important to us about persons could be stated in an impersonal way. Parfit believes that, once one accepts (3), there is not much difference between accepting (5) and (4), that is, "A person *just is* a particular brain and body, and such a series of interrelated events" (Parfit 1986, 211). Parfit's reductionism thus takes what Tännsjö calls a "deflationist" view, conceiving the notion of person in a nominalist way. "This means," according to Tännsjö, "that the notion although shallow and far from precise, plays *some* role, not in science, but in our ordinary thought in our ordinary lives. In this it is similar to the notion of something being a chair or table. We take such notions at face value. There are some clear applications of them. And it does not matter that there are borderline cases, where it is an open question whether they apply. They raise no difficult metaphysical questions. Tables and chairs are physical objects of a well-known kind." This interpretation of Parfit accords with Korsgaard's earlier remarks that metaphysical talk of persons may be innocuous if it is just talk and does not involve a commitment to, for example, Cartesian egos.

Tännsjö then suggests that one way of rescuing a notion from elimination or deflation is by theorizing. Thus, if there are good theoretical reasons for being committed to the existence of persons as all-or-nothing entities, then our inability to give a definite answer to some of the questions about personal identity raised by Parfit's hypothetical cases (e.g., his Combined Spectrum) does not imply that we should abandon persons altogether or treat them nominally. Personal identity might still involve a deep further fact beyond interrelated psychological and physical events. This further deep fact, however, need not necessarily be a Cartesian ego. It may be some other kind of theoretical entity or construct. Theorizing that persons are constituted by human organisms would be consistent with this line of thought. In the constitutive view, persons are theoretical entities posited to make sense of the varied phenomena that confront them. The constitutive theory tries to bring together in a single focus the idea that persons are biological, conscious, moral, and cultural beings.

The issue for Tännsjö is whether there is any reason to think that being a person is a deep fact. He rhetorically asks, "Does the property of being a person enter the antecedent (or consequent) of any lawlike hypotheses capable of best explaining empirical data?" In reply, he states that there is no reason to restrict the hypotheses to scientific ones and claims that the property of being a person does fit into certain *moral* hypotheses that are capable of explaining important moral data. Tännsjö argues, "If these moral hypotheses are plausible, then the fact of personal identity is indeed a deep one, or so I will argue. We should not only believe that entities that we need to have recourse to in our best (scientific) explanations of empirical data are real, we ought also to believe that entities that we need to have recourse to in our best (moral) explanations of particular moral facts (the rightness and wrongness of particular actions) are real. Metaphysically speaking, moral and scientific depth are on a par."

Tännsjö goes on to give examples of moral theories, such as egoism, theories of distributive and retributive justice, and even utilitarianism, that he believes make essential use of "the notion of being one person rather than another" and assign central importance to being able to determine where "one person's life ends and another begins." Parfit's deflationary view of persons leads to moral theories in which one's preferences about the future—for example, that Venice be saved—can be understood as a preference that some future person save Venice. The future person need not be the one with the preference. Tännsjö notes, however, that "this instrumental interest is very different from the interest presupposed in egoism that *I* be there in the future. On egoism, it is important in itself (to me) that *I* be there in the future (at least if I lead a good life; otherwise it is important that I *not* be there in the future)."

The point of reviewing Tännsjö's argument is not to favor any of the particular moral theories that assume persons as important theoretical entities for explaining moral phenomena. Rather, it is to provide further support for my claim that the concept of person is determined by considerations beyond metaphysics. I agree with Tännsjö's general claim that metaphysics and moral philosophy cannot be pursued in isolation from each other. This is particularly true with a concept such as *person*. I do not agree, however, with his claim that "moral considerations ought to determine our view of personal identity." Instead, if we are to hold in focus the various aspects that Wiggins identifies as being involved in our concept of person, we need to engage in metaphysics and moral philosophy, with an aim of achieving balance and consistency between them. The development of a mutually informed theory of personhood is the most sensible approach for dealing with the difficult cases of persons at the beginning and end of life. I have suggested that the constitutive view of persons accomplishes this better than the alternative theories.

CHAPTER EIGHT

Public Policy and the
Definition of Death

In 1999, Stuart J. Youngner, Robert M. Arnold, and Renie Schapiro published a collection of essays entitled *The Definition of Death: Contemporary Controversies.* What is perhaps most interesting about the collection is that so many of the essays reject so many of the assumptions in the current biological paradigm of death. For example, Robert Burt (1999) identifies two assumptions in the paradigm as incoherent: (1) that death is a singular determinative event rather than a process that unfolds over time and (2) that the moment of death is an objective, technologically determinable issue to which human value choices are irrelevant. Dan Brock (1999, 294) writes, "The definition of death is in part an evaluative issue, not simply a scientific question." Alta Charo (1999) starts from the assumption that the biological reality of death is "inherently ambiguous" and underdetermines the legal definition of death. According to Charo, the definition of death is more a legal fiction than a biological fact. Although some of the contributors to the volume—Robert Veatch (1999), Steven Miles (1999), and H. Tristram Engelhardt, Jr. (1999)—reject the assumptions in the biological paradigm and explicitly advocate for a more pluralistic legal definition of death, others, such as Alexander Capron (1999) and Robert Burt (1999), advocate maintaining the status quo. Burt, in fact, explicitly argues for maintaining public confidence in these beliefs, even though he acknowledges that they are intellectually indefensible.

This presents us with an interesting complication in the debate over the definition of death. Whereas some proponents of the current definition and criteria for death, such as James Bernat, believe that the assumptions in the paradigm are true (i.e., the assumptions capture the nature or reality of death), most contributors to the anthology view many of the assumptions as mistaken. Some, however, regard the assumptions as helpful fictions that should continue to be promoted by the law and medical establishment.

In this chapter, I examine whether there is any merit in maintaining public confidence in any of the assumptions of the biological paradigm even though they are groundless. In addition, should rejection of the paradigm lead to revision of the legal definition of death along more pluralistic lines that would allow individuals to choose among different criteria for death?

TRUTH OR CONSEQUENCES?

In discussing the public policy considerations concerning the definition of death, Dan Brock poses the issue as follows. Assuming that much of the public is capable of understanding many of the issues, it is "a question of whether it is better to cause public controversy and confusion up front in order to build a firmer foundation for public policy in the long run, or instead better to hide or sidestep controversy and confusion in order to achieve important policy goals in the short run" (Brock 1999, 302). Brock characterizes this choice as a choice between truth or consequences.[1]

Brock rejects what he considers the "too easy" answer that one should insist that, in public policy as in academics, we should never deviate from the truth. When it comes to public policy, he argues, truth seeking is not the only or even the most fundamental aim. Public policy must also aim at "promoting the well-being and respecting the rights of the citizens subject to that policy." He concludes, "This means that on some occasions the likely effects on the well-being and rights of the public of exposing the full complexity, ambiguity, uncertainty, and controversy surrounding a particular public policy could be sufficiently adverse and serious to justify not exposing them and presenting the issue in misleading or oversimplified terms instead" (303).

Brock is quick to note, however, that there is a very strong presumption in a democracy in favor of presenting the unvarnished truth and seeking public understanding. He also cautions against the danger of an arrogant elitism that may underlie the decisions of policymakers not to inform the public of the truth, with its ambiguities, complexities, and controversy. Nonetheless, Brock believes there is no general answer to the truth-or-consequences choices facing policymakers and that we need to weigh the specific harms and benefits involved in particular policy decisions. He does not weigh in on this issue when discussing the specific decision of whether to present the matter of defining death to the public in misleading or oversimplified terms, but he is sympathetic to the considerations that Burt has advanced for doing so.

While I think that honesty *is*, in the long run, the best public policy, let us assume that the strong presumption in favor of honest, public disclosure can sometimes be overridden by concern for the public good. We thus need to ask when this is the case and whether the definition of death is one of those cases. In my view, the presumption in favor of honest public disclosure should be overridden only when there is a serious threat of harm or loss of life to the public. For example, a government might delay the dissemination of information that would likely cause public panic, in order to take measures that would mitigate the adverse effects of the disclosure. I do not think any such serious threats of harm are of concern in the matter of defining death.

Burt, however, argues that, in the case of defining death, we should maintain the status quo "not simply in spite of its obfuscating incoherencies, but precisely because of those obfuscations" (Burt 1999, 334). He believes the obfuscations play an important role in the psychology of dying and therefore should be maintained. Thus, in support of maintaining the illusion that death is a definitive event rather than a process, Burt cites his own experience of witnessing people close to him die over a prolonged period. At some point, the progressive death was superceded by a different kind of death, a final and definitive death, at which time funeral services were held and mourning rituals were observed. "This death," he writes, "let loose feelings—of grief but of relief, of loss but of rediscovered memories—that had been in suspension during the previous prolonged slipping away." He concludes, "I can appreciate that, as an intellectual proposition, this definitive conception of death was incoherent. But as an emotional experience, it had a deeper coherence. Death conceived as a marked event permitted mourning" (335–36).

In support of maintaining a second obfuscation, that the definition of death is an objective scientific matter that is not amenable to social or individual choice, Burt believes some people would be greatly disturbed to learn that this belief is false. For them, the idea that one could choose the moment of one's death "would not only convey forbidden implications of suicide but, even more fundamentally, call into question God's independent, dispositive role in dispensing death" (336). Burt goes on to reject what he says is a standard rejoinder of pro-choice advocates in the abortion context—that is, "if you're opposed to abortion, then don't have one." He argues that this type of rejoinder has no logical application in this context, "because the opponents of choice don't simply contest those who exercise choice in dying; they deny the proposition that choice is epistemically relevant to the determination of death." Thus, allowing choice in the definition of death, according to Burt, would not be a victory for pluralism, since it would repudiate those whose values dictate that there must be only one, objective, technically dispositive definition of death. "To use the currently fashionable language of public choice theory," Burt writes, "we seem to be in a zero-sum conflict on this matter, where victory for one side constitutes total defeat for the other. In such conflicts, value pluralism cannot be vindicated. The values of some must necessarily be traversed in order to uphold the values of others" (337).

Burt goes on to suggest that, although we cannot resolve the zero-sum character of this dispute, we can evade it by taking advantage of the way patients and their proxies can legally refuse life-prolonging treatment and thereby affect the timing of death. Burt recognizes that this right to refuse treatment is not interchangeable with the right to choose a definition of death. For example, patients or proxies who wished to prolong treatment past the point when physicians are currently authorized to declare death would not be accommodated. Also, patients or proxies who wished to donate vital organs before being declared dead under the current law would not be accommodated. Burt believes, however, that, informally, some of these requests may be granted. For example, "Most hospitals are unwilling to disregard family protests to discontinue treatment modalities even if the patient meets formal criteria for the definition of death." Burt thus concludes that, because patients and their proxies can take advantage of the right to refuse treatment, those who favor revising the definition of death to allow for choice are accommodated to some degree. Thus, we better respect the values of pluralism by maintaining the status quo rather than revising the legal definition of death to allow for choice. To revise the legal definition of death in favor of choice would override the convictions of those who think that choice on this matter is disturbing and wrong. "For these latter dissenters the regime of 'choice' is an oxymoron; it is a forced choice, a paternalistic imposition that they would choose to avoid" (338).

Burt's remarks on the psychology of dying are perceptive, especially his explanation of the role that the idea of death as a definitive event rather than a process may play in allowing mourning to take place (cf. Veatch 1999). Burt never explains, however, why he accepts the idea that death is a process rather than an event. This issue was debated very early in the discussion of adopting neurological criteria for death by Leon Kass (1971) and Robert Morison (1971). According to Kass, Morison confuses the concept of death with the criteria for determining it and fails to distinguish between parts of an organism dying, which may take place gradually over time, and the death of the organism as a whole, which Kass claims to be a discrete event. Also, even if there are times when we cannot determine the moment of death, Kass argues, this does not show that death is not an event. According to Kass, in claiming that death is a process, Morison is focusing on the gradual loss of functioning of certain parts of the organism rather than what it means for the organism as a whole to cease functioning. Kass holds that, because Morison lacks a concept of the organism as a whole, he lacks an understanding of what it is that dies. In support of his claim that the "organism as a whole" is what dies, Kass refers the reader to the work of Hans Jonas. He also asserts that defining death is a medical-scientific matter and not, as Morison claims, a social-moral one.

In the same vein as Kass, James Bernat (2002, 331) criticizes those who think death is a process, such as Linda Emanuel (1995) and Halevy and Brody (1993). Bernat asserts that these theorists fail to "distinguish between our ability to determine the exact underlying state of an organism and the nature of that underlying state . . . while it may be difficult for technical reasons in some cases to determine easily or confidently whether an organism is alive or dead at a given moment, this technical limitation does not necessarily imply that the organism resides in a hypothetical in-between state" (Bernat 2002, 331). As part of the biological paradigm, Bernat holds that an organism must be in one of two states: "dead" or "alive."

Morison (1971), however, rejects the idea that death is a discrete event rather than a process, on the grounds that there is no place on the biological continuum of dying that provides a strictly biological justification for regarding it as the moment of death. Morison's point is simply that, if we regard death as a discrete moment, the justification for doing so would have to appeal to nonbiological considerations. It has nothing to do with lacking the technical resources to determine when death occurs. Morison's challenge to the claim that death is a discrete event can thus be understood as a specific challenge to the assumption in the biological paradigm that death can be defined in strictly biological terms—that is, whether we view death as an event or a process may be more a result of the values and interests that bear on our description of the biological phenomena than a result of features of the biological phenomenon itself.

While I do not think the view of death as a discrete event is "incoherent," as Burt concludes, I believe there are some problems with Kass's argument. It is odd that Kass invokes Jonas's concept of an organism in support of his claim that death is a discrete biological event. In contrast to Kass, Jonas (1974) rejected neurological criteria for death precisely because he thought that the loss of all brain function did *not* entail the loss of integration of the organism as a whole. Thus, the claim that an understanding that the organism as a whole is what dies is all one needs to recognize death as a discrete biological event, and a matter within the province of medicine or science to determine, fails to acknowledge the disagreement over what it means for an organism to exist as a whole.

Kass is right about the importance of being clear on what it is that dies, but even if we assume with Kass that what dies is the human organism, there is disagreement over what a human organism is. As noted in earlier chapters, Robert Veatch and others view the human organism as essentially a union of mind and body. In this view, the loss of consciousness and all other mental functioning would mean the loss of integration of the human organism and hence its death. Others, such as Jonas, Robert Taylor, and D. Alan Shewmon, believe that the human organism may still be integrated even if all brain function, including that of the brainstem, is lost. Still others, including Kass and Capron, claim that the human organism has necessarily lost its organic integration when all brain functions are lost. Biology cannot resolve this dispute over the nature of the human organism, since at bottom it is an issue of which characteristics are essential for human nature, and this issue extends beyond considerations of biological taxonomy. As Marx Wartofsky (1988) has pointed out, human biology is "funny biology" in the sense that values and interests inform our knowledge of the nature of a human being. Moreover, as Geertz, Callahan, and others point out, in addition to being biological animals, human beings are social-cultural beings.

If we grant Burt's claim that understanding death as a marked event is important for mourning to take place, we may wonder, does it matter for the psychology of mourning whether one is aware that viewing death as a discrete event and fixing the moment of death are the results of deliberate decision rather than biological facts? What is important for mourning may be that one understands death as a final and irreversible event. It may be irrelevant whether one thinks this event is determined by biological facts independent of choice. Even if death were a biologically discrete event independent of choice, this would not, by itself, allow mourning to take place. The person who experiences the loss must come to terms with the finality and irreversibility of death. The person has to accept that event as a mark of finality and irreversibility before mourning can take place. Thus, mourning requires an acceptance that a life is over, but this acceptance does not require a belief that no choice is involved in fixing the moment of death. In addition, it is important that such acceptance be socially reinforced, but this social reinforcement can take place regardless of whether it is true that death is a biologically discrete event.

Burt's argument that the values of pluralism are better promoted by maintaining the illusion that defining death is an objective, scientific matter, rather than one that involves choice, is also problematic for several reasons. First, this same type of zero-sum argument has been made in other contexts but is hardly persuasive. For example, Jeff Jordan (1995) has argued against the legalization of gay and lesbian marriages on the grounds that its legalization would not respect the values of those who oppose it and that the interests of gays and lesbians can be accommodated in ways short of legal recognition of their marriage. If gay and lesbian marriages were legalized, Jordan argues, the values and interests of those who oppose it would be trampled. Similar arguments were made in favor of proscribing interracial marriage. Those who think the definition and determination of death do not involve choice can live in a world in which others think there is a choice and in which they exercise that choice. Moreover, it is unclear how these people who deny choice are affected. What harm is done to them? They can continue to believe that death is an objective matter and endorse whatever criteria they believe are most consistent with their other beliefs.

Second, even if one accepted Burt's zero-sum argument that those who think that defining death does not involve choice would have their values trampled, his claim that the values and interests of those who accept that defining death does involve choice can be accommodated is questionable. While it is true that patients and, at least in some venues in the United States, their proxies can refuse life-sustaining treatment that would result in satisfying the current legal criteria for death, there are many instances in which this strategy is not an adequate accommodation. For example, respect for the "dead donor" rule precludes families from donating the vital organs of anencephalics, since anencephalics do not satisfy the current legal criteria for death.[2] If the legal criteria for death were changed to allow families to accept the irreversible loss of consciousness as death, these families would have a way of coming to terms with their loss that they currently do not have. For example, in a Florida case, the parents' request to be allowed to donate the organs of their anencephalic infant was denied by a judge on the grounds that death is a fact, not an opinion (*In re T. A. C. P.* 609 So.2d 588 [Fla. 1992]). It is hard to see how this type of court ruling, based on such a fundamental mistake about defining death, provided any accommodation to the parents' beliefs, values, and interests.

Third, Burt's claim (1999, 338) that "most hospitals are unwilling to disregard family protests to discontinue treatment modalities even if the patient meets formal criteria for the definition of death" is questionable. As noted in chapter 1, New Jersey is the only state in the United States that currently provides a statutory remedy in the form of a "conscience clause" in the legal definition of death that allows patients and families who reject neurological criteria for death to essentially opt out of having those criteria apply. New York law also allows for some discretion on the part of physicians to respect the values of patients and their families in considering the criteria for determining death. There is no accommodation, however, in these states or in any other state for allowing patients and families who accept the irreversible loss of consciousness as death to act on their beliefs. Although proponents of the consciousness-related formulation of death have not legally challenged the New Jersey and New York statutes, the statutes involve, prima facie, a violation of equal protection of the law. Why should some American Indians and Orthodox Jews who reject brain death as death be allowed to act on their beliefs, but those who accept a consciousness-related formulation of death for religious or philosophical reasons be precluded from acting on their beliefs?

Finally, while there is some evidence of hospitals continuing "life-sustaining" treatment for patients who have satisfied the neurological criteria for death, acceding to the wishes of patients and families who reject brain death as death, there are no studies confirming this practice, and I suspect that it is *not* the norm. I think what more frequently happens is that the medical paradigm simply gets imposed on families and that any reservations a family might have about whether brain death is death are never examined. Hospitals do not routinely inform patients that acceptance of neurological criteria for death may be at odds with their other beliefs or that some people do not accept brain death as death. Why complicate matters? It is much easier to simply declare death and not give patients and families a choice. Decisions about withdrawing or withholding life support can often be time-consuming and difficult. Perpetuation of the myth that defining and determining death is a strictly scientific matter may relieve patients, families, and health care providers of the burden that comes with such decision-making. If death is a biological fact, there is no choice to be made.

Relief of this burden comes with a cost, however. The cost may entail augmenting the suffering of families and disturbing the process by which they can best come to terms with loss of a loved one. Rather than facilitating mourning, determining death in a way that may conflict with families' beliefs may interfere with mourning. It may impose a directive to mourn when one is not ready to mourn, as in the case of those who, on some level, reject neurological criteria for death. For those who accept a consciousness-related formulation of death, it may prevent them from mourning even though they believe the person is gone. Their mourning must be delayed until the legal definition of death is satisfied. In addition, as the case of Nancy Cruzan illustrates, the family may face the legal and medical burdens of withdrawing life-sustaining care, such as artificial feeding and hydration. If such patients and families had the choice to accept a consciousness-related formulation of death, then the families of those who make this choice would not have to endure the hardship of watching their relative "die" by dehydration. Individuals who had irreversibly lost the capacity for consciousness would be legally dead, and a more "humane" way of terminating their remaining "vital signs," such as by lethal injection as opposed to dehydration, could be done without violating laws prohibiting euthanasia. Socially

acceptable protocols for terminating life support for individuals in a permanent vegetative state (PermVS) could be developed in the same way that we have developed
protocols for withdrawing life support from whole-brain-dead bodies.

Burt considers the United States lucky to have avoided the ideologically polariz-
ing implications of selecting the criteria for determining death that Japan has experienced. Such an assessment is too quick and easy. It is true that brain death and organ
transplantation have been extremely controversial in Japan, but this controversy orig-
inated and was exacerbated when the Japanese public became aware of several cases
of highly questionable medical practice involving the procurement of organs for
transplantation. The most infamous was the Wada case in 1968, in which a thoracic
surgeon, Dr. Wada Jiro, was charged with intentional homicide and professional neg-
ligence resulting in the death of the donor and the recipient on whom he performed
an experimental heart transplantation. It was questionable both whether the donor
was ever reliably determined to be "brain dead" and whether the recipient even required a heart transplant. Margaret Lock notes that the Wada case "set off a train of
events that made it impossible to do organ transplants making use of brain-dead
donors without serious fear of legal reprisals. It is therefore perhaps not surprising that
it has taken nearly three decades for brain death to be legally recognized in Japan, and
then only under strictly specified conditions, nor that thirty-one years passed before a
second heart transplant was carried out, in March 1999" (Lock 2002, 134).

The nearly universal public outrage in Japan over the Wada case was healthy, as
it reflected a deep concern about human rights and provided a check that social institutions must ensure those rights are respected. I would be more concerned about
a society in which the public ignored the injustice and the government swept the
matter under the rug.

Although the subsequent debate over brain death in Japan has been ideologically
divisive, it has also brought to public awareness some very important issues and challenges. First, it has made people more aware of the dangers associated with medical
experimentation and this, presumably, will help to avoid those problems in the future. After a long public debate, the Organ Transplant Law was passed in Japan in
1997. Under this law, there are rigorous standards for determining brain death, the
patient must have previously given written consent, and the family must concur
with the patient's decision.

Second, the debate has caused people to reflect more carefully on technology.
Instead of blindly accepting the technological imperative that if technology is available it must be used, the Japanese have stopped to think about the social and ethical repercussions. Some writers in Japan, such as Abe Tomoko, suggest that brain
death "transforms the process of dying into a technologically determined point in

time, as early as possible along the spectrum of biological demise" (Lock 1999, 246). Abe Tomoko is concerned that families may not easily adjust to this idea and may feel that death is being declared before the process is complete. Others point to the fact that brain death can be determined only by trained medical personnel and that this "represents a radical departure from the usual situation, where the family participates fully in the dawning recognition of the process" (Lock 1999, 246). Families are thus pushed to the sidelines and left at the mercy of medical decision-making.

Albert Borgman (1984), following Heidegger, calls attention to how technology can come between the subject and the world and can adversely mask or filter reality in ways we may fail to appreciate. The technology may provide us with some benefit—central heating, for example, may save us time and may be more convenient than feeding a wood-burning stove (Borgman's example). But we may lose worthwhile things in the process, such as familial cohesiveness promoted by daily gatherings by the fire. The Japanese seem to be much more keenly aware than many other people of how accepting brain death as death may conflict with other beliefs and how it affects their relation to loved ones. They are wrestling with a conflict between technology and their way of life. Again, this is not something that should be avoided but a challenge that should be directly addressed. Otherwise, the likely result is that technology simply rides roughshod over the beliefs and values that may be at stake.

Finally, while it is very difficult to make *any* generalizations about "Eastern" or "Western" thought, I have noted in earlier chapters that the Western philosophical tradition evinces a strong commitment to the view that at least some psychological characteristics, or the potential for some, are minimally necessary for personhood. This may not be true in the Eastern philosophical tradition. On Japanese views of personhood and brain death, Lock writes, "the person (*hito*) is not equated with individual consciousness, nor is the person located in the brain. Personhood is diffused throughout the mind and body and, moreover, is a condition that is fundamentally social and not individual in essence. An individual becomes a person only through maturation and participation in social life and ceases to be a person only after certain rituals are fulfilled" (Lock 1999, 253). If Lock is right, this may explain, at least in part, why "brain death" has been less readily accepted in Japan. If personal consciousness is not central to the Japanese idea of personhood, why would the loss of brain function be sufficient for death? In addition, by requiring the consent of the family, the Japanese Organ Transplant Law may reflect the Japanese assumption that persons are essentially social beings.

Some Japanese intellectuals have criticized brain death as too "unnatural" (*fushizen*) to be equated with death (Lock 1997). This is perhaps consistent with Robert Veatch's and Karen Gervais's point that it is wrong to think of the irreversible loss of brain function as simply a new way of determining when death, as tradition-ally understood, occurs. Veatch and Gervais believe that acceptance of brain death as death entails a conceptual shift to the irreversible loss of consciousness as a new meaning of death. They might agree with these Japanese intellectuals that brain death does represent a new way of dying, an "unnatural" way brought about by ad-vances in medical technology. Although those who accept the biological paradigm of death assume that there cannot be any new ways of dying (David Lamb [1985], for example, is quite explicit about this), I agree with Veatch and Gervais. Thus, there is an interesting twist. The Japanese intellectuals who have criticized brain death as unnatural are forthright in recognizing what is at stake by accepting brain death — namely, that we are classifying a new, technologically created type of phenomenon as death. This is unacceptable to some Japanese people because it challenges their reluctance to view personal consciousness as central to personal existence. Western-ers, by contrast, operate with the illusion that the irreversible loss of all brain func-tions is simply a new criterion for determining when death, as traditionally under-stood, occurs. What really makes brain death acceptable in the West, however, is not this illusion but that brain death is a new way in which people can suffer an irre-versible loss of consciousness, which Westerners are willing to accept as the end of personal existence (i.e., death). This argues for taking a pluralistic approach to defin-ing death. Here, I agree with Lock's conclusion that the lesson to be learned from the Japanese experience is that, "in this transnational world of increasingly pluralistic so-cieties, we must begin to recognize a multiplicity of ways of comprehending and le-galizing the process of dying and the management of the death" (Lock 1999, 253).

IF IT'S BROKE, FIX IT

The 1981 President's Commission for the Study of Ethical Problems in Medicine and Biomedical and Behavioral Research maintains that "brain-based criteria do not introduce a new 'kind of death,' but rather reinforce the concept of death as a single phenomenon—the collapse of psycho-physical integrity. The statute merely allows new ways to recognize that this phenomenon has occurred" (President's Commission 1981, 58). In the very next paragraph of the report, however, under the heading "Death of the Organism as a Whole," the commission states, "The death of the human being—not the 'death' of cells, tissues, or organism—is the matter at issue" (58). These lines reveal a basic ambiguity or contradiction in identifying what the commission was trying to propose criteria for. Was the commission's intent to propose a new way of determining the point of (1) collapse of psychophysical in-tegrity or (2) death of the human organism as a whole? These phenomena are different. If *psycho* refers to mentality or psychological functions of any sort in the expression "psychophysical integrity," the irreversible loss of consciousness, sentience, and every other mental function is sufficient for a collapse of psychophysical integrity, even if it is not sufficient for the loss of integration of the organism as a whole. Also, as pointed out in earlier chapters, cases of postmortem pregnancy and the extraordinary case reported by Shewmon (1998b) in which a whole-brain-dead patient was sustained for more than fourteen years challenge the underlying assumption that brain function is necessary for organic integration. It is simply no longer plausible to maintain that human organisms that have lost all brain function cannot be "integrated" as a whole.

At the time of the report of the President's Commission, there were no cases in which whole-brain-dead human organisms could be sustained for such lengthy time frames. As the commission acknowledges,

> A more significant criticism [of the whole-brain formulation] shares the view that life consists of the coordinated functioning of the various bodily systems, in which process the whole-brain plays a crucial role. At the same time, it notes that in some adult patients lacking all brain functions it is possible through intensive support to achieve constant temperature, metabolism, waste disposal, blood pressure, and other conditions typical of living organisms and not found in dead ones. Even with extraordinary medical care, these functions cannot be sustained indefinitely—typically no longer than several days—but it is argued that this shows only that patients with nonfunctional brains are dying, not that they are dead. In this view, the respirator, drugs, and other resources of the modern intensive-care unit collectively substitute for the lower brain, just as a pump used in cardiac surgery takes over the heart's function. (President's Commission 1981, 35)

The commission tried to dismiss this objection by claiming, implausibly, that what remains in such a case with artificial medical support is "merely a group of artificially maintained subsystems." This claim is implausible because it fails to explain why the loss of autonomous regulation by the brain is so significant for the maintenance of the human organism as a whole. Just as we think a human organism's dependence on artificial life support in other circumstances does not entail the organism's loss of its organic integration, there is no reason to think that, because the regulative functions of the brainstem are taken over by artificial means, there is no longer an integrated human organism. In fact, in the case of brain-dead pregnant women, there is so much integration that another life (that of the fetus) can be sustained.

In addition, Shewmon (2004b) has critiqued the claim that brain function is necessary for the maintenance of organic integration in organisms with a brain, by comparing the somatic state of whole-brain-dead individuals with that of patients who have sustained high spinal cord transection, resulting in the irreversible loss of spontaneous respiration, cardiovascular activity, temperature control, and other integrating functions.[3] Shewmon demonstrates that these two types of conditions are somatically similar with respect to the loss of integrative functions. Thus, if we do not think high cord transection results in the irreversible loss of organic integration in a human organism and that the human organism has therefore died, there is no reason to think the loss of all brain functions has this result. Shewmon thus undermines the standard rationale for accepting the loss of all brain functions as death.

Shewmon points out that his argument only has implications for the conceptual validity of the *biological rationale* for accepting the loss of all brain functions as a criterion for death. He acknowledges that his argument does not address the alternative rationale for adopting neurological criteria for determining death that has been offered by proponents of a consciousness-related formulation of death. As indicated in earlier chapters, by distinguishing the death of the person from that of the organism, a consciousness-related formulation can consistently maintain that a person has died, even though an integrated human organism may persist. I have suggested that we have been willing to accept brain death as death not because we have been certain that it constitutes the irreversible loss of organic integration but because we have been certain that it entails the irreversible loss of consciousness and every other mental function—that is, it entails the collapse of our "psychophysical integrity."

If the biological paradigm is broken but we think that brain function is essential to our being the kind of beings that we are, the first step is to put acceptance of neurological criteria for determining death on firmer conceptual grounds. These grounds have been available all along but have been rejected for the wrong reasons. As mentioned in chapter 1, one of the reasons why the President's Commission and others rejected the personhood argument for a consciousness-related definition of death was that they rejected what they thought was an implication of the definition: that it would entail treating individuals in a persistent vegetative state as dead. They also were concerned that it would lead down a slippery slope: "Severely senile patients, for example, might not clearly be persons, let alone ones with continuing personal identities; the same might be true of the severely retarded. Any argument that classified these individuals as dead would not meet with public acceptance" (President's Commission 1981, 40).

The commission offers no rationale for its concern. If the consensus about persons that underlies acceptance of neurological criteria for death is only that persons must minimally have the capacity or potential for consciousness and does not involve discriminating among different mental capacities or potentials, then there is

no threat to the severely senile or severely retarded. Since individuals in these conditions suffer dementia, not amentia, the consciousness-related definition of death
does not rule them out of the class of persons and hence provides no reason for considering them to be dead. In short, there is no slippery slope.

Acceptance of a consciousness-related formulation of death does not entail anything about the specific neurological criteria that should be used, as a practical matter, to determine death. The President's Commission questioned whether adequate
medical techniques are currently available to implement this formulation:

> In order to be incorporated into public policy, a conceptual formulation of death has
> to be amenable to clear articulation. At present, neither basic neurophysiology nor
> medical technique suffices to translate the "higher-brain" formulation into policy.
> First . . . it is not known which portions of the brain are responsible for cognition and
> consciousness; what little is known points to substantial interconnections among the
> brainstem, subcortical structures and the neocortex. Thus, the "higher brain" may well
> exist only as a metaphorical concept, not in reality. Second, even when the sites of cer-
> tain aspects of consciousness can be found, their cessation often cannot be assessed
> with the certainty that would be required in applying a statutory definition. (President's
> Commission 1981, 40)

This argument expresses a concern about implementing a consciousness-related
formulation—about whether there are adequate means for determining when an irreversible loss of consciousness has occurred. It says nothing about whether that formulation is acceptable. As Veatch has pointed out, the commission's concern "may
lead to the policy conclusion that in order to pronounce people dead (based on
higher-brain conceptualizations of death) we must revert to the old whole-brain oriented criteria. The logic of such a move is that persons will be considered dead when
they lose higher-brain function, but that the only way we can know for sure that
higher-brain function has been lost is to demonstrate that all brain function has been
lost." Veatch's point is that, although the argument may lead to the conclusion that,
for policy purposes alone, we should not at this time distinguish whole-brain from
higher-brain criteria for determining death, "the decision is surely not a sound argument against the position that people ought to be considered dead when it can be
determined that they have irreversibly lost higher-brain function" (Veatch 1988, 177).

PERSISTENT AND PERMANENT VEGETATIVE STATES

Ronald Cranford (1988) details the diagnostic and prognostic complexities surrounding the persistent vegetative state (PVS), the condition often cited as repre-

sentative of a complete, irreversible loss of consciousness. Cranford's remarks are as true today as when he wrote them. If anything, the diagnostic and prognostic complexities have increased in the light of recent studies. "For several reasons," Cranford writes, "the degree of certainty about diagnosis of this syndrome is less absolute than a diagnosis of brain death." He continues:

> With the persistent vegetative state . . . there is no broadly accepted set of specific medical criteria with as much clinical detail and certainty as the brain death criteria. Furthermore, even the generally accepted criteria, when properly applied, are not infallible. There have been a few unexpected, but unequivocal and well documented, recoveries of cognitive functions in situations where it was believed that the criteria were correctly applied by several neurologists experienced in the diagnosis of the condition. In cases in New Mexico and Minnesota, the patients recovered full cognitive functioning, although they were left with a severe and permanent paralysis of all extremities and some paralysis of facial and head movements, i.e., locked-in syndrome . . .
>
> Presently, there are no specific laboratory studies to confirm the clinical diagnosis of the persistent vegetative state. After a variable period of time (weeks to months), some studies such as MRI [magnetic resonance imaging] and CAT (computerized axial tomography) scanning will show extensive structural damage to the cerebral hemispheres consistent with the clinical diagnosis but these studies are not quantifiable. The most promising test on the horizon that will be of value in confirming a clinical diagnosis of the persistent vegetative state is the PET (positron emission tomography scan) . . .
>
> The electroencephalogram (EEG) also does not provide absolute certainty because the degree of abnormality of the EEG will vary widely in individual cases. Some appear remarkably normal considering the extent of damage to the cerebral hemispheres . . .
>
> Prognostic assessments of patients in a persistent vegetative state are not free of controversy. A major problem is attributable to the multiple causes and pathophysiologic changes associated with the syndrome. In brain death, the underlying cause of the brain injury is not so important once the basic sequence of pathophysiologic events begins and lead inexorably to its conclusion (severe primary injury—brain swelling—marked increase in intracranial pressure—increased intracranial pressure exceeding blood pressure, causing secondary loss of blood flow to the entire brain—infarction of cerebral hemispheres and the brain stem). In the persistent vegetative state, however, there are multiple causes for the syndrome, and no single pathophysiologic sequence of events. Therefore, the prognosis of recovery of neurological function, when the prognosis can be made, and its degree of certainty will vary considerably according to the underlying cause of the brain damage and the specific pathophysiology. (Cranford 1988, 29–30)[4]

In 1994, the Multi-Society Task Force on PVS (MSTF), an illustrious group of neurologists, pediatricians, and neurosurgeons, issued a consensus statement summarizing the current knowledge of the medical aspects of the persistent vegetative state in adults and children. The report of the MSTF was endorsed by the American Academy of Neurology, American Neurological Association, American Association of Neurological Surgeons, and Child Neurology Society. The report states,

> The vegetative state is a clinical condition of complete unawareness of the self and the environment, accompanied by sleep-wake cycles, with either complete or partial preservation of hypothalamic and brain-stem autonomic functions. In addition, patients in a vegetative state show no evidence of sustained, reproducible, purposeful, or voluntary behavioral responses to visual, auditory, tactile, or noxious stimuli; show no evidence of language comprehension or expression; have bowel and bladder incontinence; and have variably preserved cranial-nerve and spinal reflexes. We define persistent vegetative states as a vegetative state present one month after acute traumatic or nontraumatic brain injury or lasting for at least one month in patients with degenerative or metabolic disorders or developmental malformations . . .
>
> Recovery of consciousness from a posttraumatic persistent vegetative state is unlikely after 12 months in adults and children. Recovery from a nontraumatic persistent vegetative state after three months is exceedingly rare in both adults and children. (MSTF 1994, 1499)

The report of the MSTF has been criticized as conceptually confused (Howsepian 1996; Borthwick 1996; Shewmon 1997, 2004a) on two main grounds. First, critics argue that the MSTF mistakenly takes the absence of evidence for consciousness as evidence for the absence of consciousness. Patients in locked-in syndrome, for example, are unable to communicate that they are conscious, other than by blinking their eyes in response to questioning. Suppose these patients were unable to signal by blinking their eyes. It would be a mistake to infer that they lacked consciousness. Given the similarities in the evidence used to diagnose both conditions, critics argue that there is no way to tell for certain whether the individual in PVS lacks consciousness. As Shewmon (1997, 60) suggests, individuals in PVS may be in a "super-locked-in" state. Howsepian (1994, 752) suggests that "there actually may be something that it is like to be comatose."

The second main criticism challenges the warrant for calling some PVS cases "permanent," as the MSTF admits it is possible, although highly unlikely, that someone in a permanent vegetative state might recover. The possibility of recovery seems to contradict the meaning of "permanent."

There is some merit to these criticisms. The report certainly could have been more careful in its language to avoid some of the conceptual inconsistencies that are pounced upon by its critics, especially Howsepian (1996). I think the critics err, however, in what seems to be their demand for absolute certainty in the diagnosis of a lack of consciousness in PVS and the prognosis of permanency. Neither demand can be met, but that should not discount the usefulness of PVS and PermVS as, respectively, diagnostic and prognostic categories. Although at one point Howsepian (1994) cites some passages from Aristotle's *Nicomachean Ethics* to support a claim about virtuous conduct toward comatose individuals, he seems to ignore Aristotle's advice that we should not expect more precision than the subject matter admits (*Nicomachean Ethics* 1.3.1094b10–15).

The first criticism essentially relies on a claim about the impossibility of knowing whether another being is conscious, what in philosophy is called the "problem of other minds." Since we seem to have direct access only to the contents of our own minds, how can we know for sure whether there are any other minds?[5] Moreover, since it is clearly possible that someone might be conscious without exhibiting behavior that indicates their consciousness (just as the Spartan may be in severe pain but not exhibit any pain behavior), we cannot infer from the absence of behavioral evidence of consciousness that there is no consciousness (Putnam 1980). As Shewmon (2004a, 222) states, "the lack of 'behavioral indication' of any awareness of pain or suffering [in cases of PVS] does not *per se* imply a lack of pain or suffering." Alternatively, someone might exhibit what we normally recognize as pain behavior but not be in pain. Thus, the grunting, grimacing, groaning, avoidance movements, and so forth, that individuals in PVS sometimes exhibit are standardly interpreted as stereotypical, unconscious reflexive responses. Shewmon asks, however, "On what plausible ground can anyone confidently dismiss such behaviors as invariably *not* reflecting discomfort or pain?" (225).

The diagnostic and prognostic problems associated with PVS certainly argue for a tutioristic approach in declaring dead every individual that satisfies the generally accepted criteria for a diagnosis of PVS. It is better to treat these individuals as living persons if we cannot determine with a very high degree of clinical certainty that they have irreversibly lost consciousness. The critical issue is how tutioristic we should be. Howsepian advocates that "some purportedly irreversibly comatose humans ought to be kept alive indefinitely." He does not indicate, however, where a line should be drawn between this claim and the claim that "*all* comatose humans should be kept alive indefinitely" (Howsepian 1994, 735). Should the philosophical problem of other minds commit us to keeping all individuals in PVS alive indefinitely because we cannot determine with absolute certainty that they have irreversibly lost consciousness?

I do not think so. P. F. Strawson's argument ([1958] 1991; 1959) was endorsed in chapter 4 as a reason for considering persons as a primitive kind of substance in our ontology. Strawson's argument, which perhaps can be traced back to Wittgenstein (1953), is that, to ascribe states of consciousness to ourselves, we must be able to ascribe them to others.[6] In order to ascribe them to others, however, we need to identify other subjects of experience, which is done not by observation of their inner mental states but by observation of their bodies and behavior. I consider Strawson's argument to be a partial solution to the problem of other minds, although his view is not without its difficulties.[7] What makes the problem of other minds so intolerable is that it challenges our ability to know whether any other being is conscious. This is bad enough. But if we cannot know whether any other being is conscious, then, in principle, we cannot rule out consciousness in any being. This implication is worse. Clearly, we have more reason for thinking that a normal human being is conscious than is a cake of soap or a plant. Thus, acceptance of the implications of the problem of other minds is incompatible with an empirical theory that commits us to the view that some kinds of physical beings are more likely than others to have consciousness. The question of whether any being is conscious must therefore be addressed within the context of a theory about the connection between the mind and body. Strawson lays the foundation for such a connection by establishing that we could not identify our own mental states as our own without identifying those of others on the basis of physical criteria. Neurophysiological and behavioral psychology are built on the assumption that psychology is dependent on, though perhaps not reducible to, the body. Dependency but nonreducibility may prevent Strawson's view from sliding into an untenable form of logical or ontological behaviorism. Further inquiry and theorizing about this dependency also enables us to make reasonable judgments about when consciousness is present.

Thus, the diagnostic and prognostic problems associated with PVS do not support a tutioristic line in all cases of PVS. Cranford's statement (1988), reflected in the report of the MSTF, that "the degree of certainty [of the prognosis for neurological recovery] will vary considerably according to the underlying cause of brain damage and the specific pathophysiology" suggests that, in some cases, the certainty of the prognosis may be quite high or at least higher than in other cases. If we are justified in making such comparative judgments about the presence or absence of consciousness, then the philosophical problem of other minds loses its relevancy. Since the implication of the problem of other minds is that we have no reason to think another being is conscious or unconscious, comparative judgments about the likelihood of consciousness in different physical beings would also be groundless.

Although Cranford does not elaborate on what specifically affects this degree of certainty—that is, which causes of brain damage and specific pathophysiology yield a higher degree of prognostic certainty—studies of some PVS patients' EEG activity, cerebral blood circulation, and duration of survival yield a very high degree of prognostic certainty. For example, some long-surviving (up to seventeen years) patients with apallic syndrome (i.e., with the type of unresponsiveness characteristic of PVS) studied by Ingvar and colleagues (1978) showed, over many years, repeated isoelectric EEGs and extremely low supratentorial blood flow (about 10 to 20 percent of the normal level), indicating the reduced metabolic demand of gliotic scar tissue. Despite exceptional cases of recovery from PVS, I think few neurologists would recognize a realistic potential for regaining consciousness in Ingvar's patients. Thus, while further studies of PVS patients are needed to arrive at covering laws concerning the diagnosis and prognosis of this class of cases, some individual cases can be diagnosed and prognosticated with a high degree of certainty.

Of course, a consensus among neurologists does not imply that their view is correct. Shewmon (2004a) has challenged the widely held assumption in neurology that cortical function is absolutely necessary for consciousness in terms of adaptive interaction with the environment and a subjective awareness of self and environment. Shewmon and two colleagues (1999) report having studied several cases of children with congenital apallia (loss of the pallium, or gray-matter mantle of the brain) who nonetheless clearly demonstrated conscious awareness. These children were able to hear without an auditory cortex, see without a visual cortex, and feel without a somatosensory cortex. Shewmon concludes, "Cases like these seriously undermine the concept of 'apallic syndrome' or 'neocortical death,' understood as anything beyond neuropathology, because they unequivocally prove that the absence of cortex does not necessarily result in what is generally understood as VS [vegetative state]" (Shewmon 2004a, 218).

Shewmon considers whether these cases of congenital apallia imply anything for cases of acquired apallia, such as those studied by Ingvar. He notes that patients with the acquired disorder suffer greater motor impairment than the children. He believes this should make us cautious about attributing the difference between acquired and congenital apallia entirely to a difference in the degree of brainstem plasticity for consciousness, for the difference may be due to a plasticity for motor function. Thus, according to Shewmon, "What the congenital cases imply about acquired VS in older patients is to suggest a plausible alternative to the cortex-consciousness dogma. It has never been scientifically ruled out (nor can it be), that some (unknowable number of) acquired-apallia patients have a limited form of consciousness but simply cannot manifest it due to extreme motoric disability" (218).

He goes on to note that, as is well known, the neuroanatomical pathways of pain sensation involve mainly subcortical areas. Some stroke patients may report the raw sensation of pain but not its affective component: they still feel the pain "just as before" but it "no longer bothers them" (219). Shewmon reasons that, if the necessary and apparently sufficient pathways for the sensation of pain abstracted from the affective component are intact in both congenitally and postnatally acquired apallia, "there is no reason to assume that apallia precludes all experience of pain and discomfort. The hydranencephalic children described above clearly experienced pain, as do newborns and fetuses with relatively non-functioning cortices. Therefore, when adult or older children with similar acquired lesions withdraw limbs, grimace and cry to noxious stimuli, on what grounds can anyone assert that these responses are '*merely* primitive reflexes,' even if the motor reaction is simple and stereotyped?" (219).[8]

Shewmon is on firmer ground here than when he claimed that individuals who have lost all brain function, including that of the brainstem, still have the potential for consciousness, intellect, and will. As I argued in chapter 5, Shewmon relied on an unrealistic notion of potentiality to support his claim. The children with congenital apallia provide evidence not just of the potential for consciousness but of actual consciousness without cortical structures. He does not appeal simply to the fact that individuals with congenital and acquired apallia are members of the human species to support his claim that they have the capacity for consciousness. He appeals to the fact that they are members of the human species with intact functioning brainstems and that the behavior exhibited by the congenital apallics is evidence of consciousness. If we do not know enough about PVS to rule out the possibility that the inability of individuals in this state to express their capacity for consciousness may be due to an extreme motor disability rather than a lack of capacity for consciousness, then it is *possible* that individuals in even long-term PVS retain the capacity for consciousness and therefore have not died.

Whether this is the most reasonable hypothesis, however, is unclear. In other words, even though we may not be able to rule out the possibility that these individuals have some rudimentary consciousness, it is not clear that this is a more plausible explanation than their behavior being merely reflexive and that the degree of probability of the hypothesis is sufficient to justify treating them tutioristically. Also unclear is what to make of the reports by some stroke patients that they have the raw sensation of pain minus its affective component. Without the conscious affective component, should we consider these patients to be "in pain" or suffering? If they are not in pain and are not suffering, what ethical weight should we assign to such experiences?

I have argued that a realistic potential for consciousness is a minimal necessary condition for something to be a living person. I do not know whether an organism capable of having a "raw sensation" is conscious. The "raw sensation" might be analogous to the kind of pupillary reflex discussed in the following exchange between Douglas Walton (1980) and Roland Puccetti (1988). Walton maintains that feeling and sensation may be possible even in the absence of cortical functions. For example, considering the pupillary reflex mediated by the brainstem, Walton writes, "The pupillary reflex could, for all we know, indicate some presence of feeling or sensation even if the higher cognitive faculties are absent. Even if we cannot resolve the issue with the precision that we would like and, indeed, just because of that, we should be on the safe side . . . Following my tutiorist line of argument, it is clear that we cannot rule out the possibility that brain-stem reflexes could indicate some form of sensation or feeling, even if higher mental activity is not present" (Walton 1980, 69). Walton's view, Puccetti claims,

> fairly reeks of superstition. As we all know, when the doctor flashed his penlight on the eye, we do not feel the pupil contract, then expand when he turns the light off. If not, then why in the world does Walton suppose that a deeply comatose patient feels anything in the same testing situation? The whole point of evolving reflexes like this, especially in large brained animals that do little peripheral but lots of central information processing, is to shunt quick-response mechanisms away from the cerebrum so that the animal can make appropriate initial responses to stimuli *before* registering them consciously. If one could keep an excised human eye alive *in vitro* and provoke the pupillary reflex, the way slices of rat hippocampus have been stimulated to threshold for neuronal excitation, would Walton argue that the isolated eye might feel something as the pupil contracts? (Puccetti 1988, 78)

I agree with Puccetti that it is unreasonable to think the pupillary reflex necessarily involves consciousness. If the raw sensations of the stroke victim and the stereotypical behavior exhibited by some individuals in PVS are similar to the pupillary reflex, then it is implausible to think these "sensations" or behavior involve conscious awareness.

Critics of extending the consciousness-related formulation of death to anencephalics and individuals in PVS also raise issues about the diagnostic reliability of these conditions (Shewmon 1988, 2004a; Capron 1987). Shewmon, for example, states, "In a great majority of cases, the diagnosis of anencephaly is very obvious, and there is little chance of mistaking it for another condition. Nevertheless, not all cases are so straightforward. If anencephaly were clearly distinct from all other congenital brain malformations, it should be possible to give an operational definition of it that includes all cases of anencephaly and excludes cases of everything else, yet such a definition has not been offered by anyone so far" (Shewmon 1988, 11–12). He goes on to give examples of diagnostic ambiguity between anencephaly ("a partial or total absence of the brain") and other less severe congenital malformations: exencephaly ("exposure of the brain"), encephaloceles ("hernias of the brain protruding through a congenital opening of the skull"), meroanencephaly or meroacrania ("a partial absence of brain and calvarium [calvaria]"), and amniotic band syndrome ("a broad continuum of severity that can mimic anencephaly").

Shewmon's point is that these cases constitute a spectrum of neural organization and, in some cases, it is impossible to distinguish one condition from another. Individuals that fall at the less-developed end of the spectrum, such as anencephalics, clearly have no cerebral tissue and thus no cerebral function. Individuals at the other end of the spectrum, such as meroanencephalics, have some rudimentary cerebral tissue and therefore may have some cerebral function — for example, they may be capable of suffering. Shewmon concludes, "These examples are not intended to exaggerate the potential for diagnostic confusion surrounding anencephaly: it is still quite true that in the vast majority of cases the diagnosis can be made easily and without risk of error. Nevertheless, the commonly encountered contention that 'anencephaly' is so well defined and distinct from all other congenital brain malformations that misdiagnosis cannot occur and that organ harvesting policies limited to 'anencephalics' cannot possibly extend to other conditions, is simply false" (12).

In the case of PVS, the possibility of misdiagnosis is more troublesome. Keith Andrews and colleagues (1996) report that, in their study of forty patients referred to as being in a persistent vegetative state, seventeen (43%) were misdiagnosed. Seven of these misdiagnosed patients had been presumed to be vegetative for more than one year, including three for longer than four years. Similar findings of misdiagnosis (an error rate of 37%) are reported by Childs, Mercer, and Childs, who conclude that the error in diagnosis may result from "confusion in terminology, lack of extended observation of patients, and lack of skill or training in the assessment of neurologically devastated patients" (Childs et al. 1993, 1465).

More recently, Giacino and colleagues (2002) have proposed defining and establishing diagnostic criteria for the minimally conscious state (MCS). They define MCS as "a condition of severely altered consciousness in which minimal but definite behavioral evidence of self or environmental awareness is demonstrated" (350–51). Patients in MCS have "neurologic findings that do not meet criteria for VS [vegetative state]. These patients demonstrate discernible behavioral evidence of consciousness but remain unable to reproduce this behavior consistently . . . MCS is distinguished from VS by the partial preservation of conscious awareness" (349–50).

This alternative diagnosis may be helpful in distinguishing cases of severe brain injury in which some conscious recovery is possible. Joseph Fins explains,

> Recent studies have shown . . . that patients can regain some evidence of consciousness before the vegetative state becomes permanent. In the window between the persistent and permanent vegetative state, patients can progress to what has been described as the "minimally conscious state" (MCS). Unlike vegetative patients, the minimally conscious demonstrate unequivocal, but fluctuating evidence of awareness of self and environment. The natural history of MCS is not yet known. Near the upper boundary of this category, patients may say words or phrases and gesture. They may also show evidence of memory, attention, and intention. Patients are considered to have "emerged" from MCS only when they can reliably and consistently communicate. (Fins 2005, 22)

Fins is quick to point out that, although "recent studies suggest that the diagnostic distinction between MCS and PVS is missed by neurologists at rates that would be intolerable in other clinical domains," we should not conclude that there is no distinction between these conditions or between PVS and PermVS (22; cf. Schiff and Fins 2003). In the highly publicized case of Terri Schiavo in Florida, Fins is critical of the kind of diagnostic distortion used by some for political ends. "In Schiavo," he writes, "right to life advocates asserted that she was not vegetative. By suggesting consciousness where there was none, these opponents of choice at the end of life cast doubt on the ethical propriety of removing life-sustaining therapy. They persisted even though court-appointed physicians found that she was vegetative, and even when the Florida Supreme Court determined that there was clear and convincing evidence for this diagnosis" (Fins 2005, 23). Fins and Plum caution, "while a diverse society can ascribe different meaning to life in a permanent vegetative state, these valuations should not undermine an accurate diagnosis nor falsely suggest that recovery of consciousness from the permanent vegetative state is possible. Such misinformation—often the product of journalistic excess—engenders false expectations by erroneously suggesting that the permanent vegetative are capable of recovery" (Fins and Plum 2004, 1354). At the same time that Fins and Plum stress the need to identify patients with some potential for recovery and provide them with emerging rehabilitative strategies, they caution against offering false hope to others who are "beyond the reach of any hope known to science" (1355). The need for careful neurological assessment is obviously critical. The frequency of misdiagnosis should not lead to the conclusion that PVS and PermVS can never be accurately diagnosed.[9]

As noted above, the problems associated with the diagnosis of anencephaly and PVS do not challenge the consciousness-related formulation of death. They do, however, raise issues about whether we could reliably implement a policy of determining death that would include anencephalics and individuals in PermVS. Shinnar and Arras (1989, 730) point out that, in the vast majority of cases, the diagnosis of anencephaly can be reliably made and there is little chance of mistaking it for another condition. Shewmon concurs (1988, 12). Shewmon's study, however, although including only three children, raises issues about the potential for consciousness in anencephalics. Further study is needed to determine whether the consciousness that his patients exhibited is possible for all anencephalics or whether we can make reliable discriminations about the presence or absence of the potential for consciousness in infants diagnosed with anencephaly.

There is less diagnostic certainty and reliability about PVS. Again, for the purpose of satisfying a consciousness-related formulation of death, the critical determination is whether these individuals have a potential for consciousness. The Multi-Society Task Force concluded that data on the prognosis for neurological recovery of patients in PVS, "in conjunction with other relevant factors in an individual patient, can be used by a physician to determine when the persistent vegetative state becomes permanent—that is, when a physician can tell the patient's family or surrogate with a high degree of medical certainty that there is no further hope for recovery of consciousness or that, if consciousness were recovered, the patient would be left severely disabled" (MSTF 1994, 1501).

It is unfortunate that the MSTF conflates the notion of what it means for the loss of consciousness to be "permanent" and the possibility of recovery of consciousness with severe disability. If the caveat about the possibility of recovery is simply an expression of the MSTF's recognition that all diagnoses in medicine are based on probabilities and not certainty, then the qualification is innocuous. If absolute certainty were required before implementing a medical policy for determining death, no medical policy could ever be implemented. As Norman Fost points out in the context of his discussion of anencephaly, "not all clinicians or hospitals would be equally competent at making the diagnosis and errors have occurred with anencephaly, just as they have occurred with the simpler (or easier) diagnosis of brain death" (Fost 1988, 8).

If, however, the MSTF were expressing greater reservations about the clinical certainty of the diagnosis of permanent loss of consciousness, then reliance on a diagnosis of permanent vegetative state to satisfy a consciousness-related definition of death would be more problematic. This is why, at the outset of this work, I stipulated that I was using the term *permanent vegetative state* (PermVS) to mean a vegetative state in which the probability of regaining consciousness is extremely remote — beyond what I defined (when discussing Shewmon's views in chapter 5) as "realistic probability." I believe this standard can be met for some individuals in PVS, such as the long-surviving individuals studied by Ingvar. Thus, while the diagnostic and prognostic uncertainty about PVS would argue against allowing the diagnosis to satisfy a consciousness-related formulation of death, there are some cases of PermVS that could reliably be said to satisfy the formulation. Clearly, further work on PVS must be done to develop finer criteria for distinguishing it from other conditions and to identify more clearly those factors in the syndrome itself and in individual patients that contribute to making the condition permanent and irreversible.

A PLURALISTIC PROPOSAL

Since the start of debate over the legal definition of death, there has been disagreement about whether *death* should be defined uniformly among people and situations. The 1981 President's Commission considered Roger Dworkin's proposal (1973) that, instead of asking the question "what is death?" we should ask, "what difference does it make whether somebody is dead?" Dworkin suggests that the latter question has many different answers, depending on the context, and that we should legally recognize different definitions of death for different purposes. Dworkin thinks it would be odd if a single definition of death sufficed to resolve all the situations that depend on a definition of death for their resolution.[10]

Dworkin's proposal is further developed by Susan Brennan and Richard Delgado in their exploration of the implications of adopting a contextual, or functional, approach to defining death. They suggest that "the question 'Is x dead?' is answered differently depending on the purpose for which the question is asked and the consequences that flow from the answer" (Brennan and Delgado 1981, 1324). They examine three areas of law (double indemnity life insurance, autopsy and burial, and organ transplantation) and propose that different physical definitions of death be adopted in each area. In double indemnity insurance, for example, they observe that time limitation clauses, originally designed to ensure proof of causation in accident cases, have become less useful with medical advances that permit doctors to control the timing of death. In this context, they suggest, consideration of the interests of the victims and families warrant adopting a higher-brain formulation of death. In contrast, they argue that, for purposes of autopsy and burial, we should define death in terms of the cessation of circulatory and respiratory functions rather than loss of brain function.

The Organ Transplant Law in Japan adopts this multiple-standard approach. Brain death is equated with death *only* for the purposes of organ donation. Margaret Lock suggests that the law "signifies formal recognition of something like the 'alpha period' suggested by Bai Koichi nearly thirty years earlier, an ambiguous time of living death to which special laws can be applied" (Lock 2002, 181). As Lock explains, Bai Koichi, a lawyer,

> recognized that "the body may for a while show features of both life and death," after "death of the brain." He suggests that this time could be called the "alpha period," a time that lies "between life and death, but belonging to neither." In Bai's opinion, a legal agreement could be hammered out specifically to cover the removal of organs during the alpha period, provided that potential donors have given prior assent and close relatives agree. Bai is sensitive to the fact that all existing law in connection with life and death depends on a dichotomous distinction. He insists that such a distinction is in effect, arbitrary, although he recognizes its utility in law; but he believes that some flexibility is in order when it comes to the new technological death. (136)[11]

Bai's "alpha period" is similar to Dworkin's view that death is a process that is sometimes prolonged and that different stages in the process might be considered to constitute death for different purposes (see also Emanuel 1995). In another respect, however, Bai's approach and the Japanese Organ Transplant Law go further than the proposals by Dworkin, Brennan, and Delgado. Bai and the Japanese law provide for the potential donor and relatives to choose brain death as the criterion for determining death in the context of organ transplantation. The law does not simply state that brain death may be used as a criterion for determining death in all cases in which organ donation may be possible. Rather, it makes acceptance of this criterion dependent on decisions by the donor and relatives. The proposals by Dworkin, Brennan, and Delgado may allow for this type of individual choice in the legal definition of death, but it is not clear that they appreciate how the values of respect for autonomy, family decision-making, and pluralism may mandate it. For example, on the question of which definition of death should be used in the context of organ donation, Brennan and Delgado suggest three alternatives: (1) adopt a single, early, whole- or part-brain standard, (2) allow the donor or next of kin to choose the standard that he or she wishes to have applied, and (3) allow the physician to choose the standard to apply (Brennan and Delgado 1981, 1354). Alternatives (1) and (3) do not adequately recognize the values of autonomy, family decision-making, pluralism, and specific cultural conditions that can be used to support option (2), which is what the Japanese law has done.

Fost (1999) has recently tried to expand on the position of Dworkin, Brennan, and Delgado by suggesting that a definition of death is not necessary to address the various issues that we thought required one. He thinks we would be better off if we had not expanded the legal criteria for determining death to include neurological criteria and, instead, had chosen to address the issues by relevant moral and legal considerations. "The social purposes for declaring a patient dead (e.g., cessation of treatment, organ removal, settling estates, burial, etc.) can be justified in other ways. It was and is not necessary to conclude that a patient is dead to accomplish those social goals in a morally and legally satisfactory way" (Fost 1999, 161).

Fost considers, for example, whether the move to a neurological criterion of death has helped or hindered organ donation: "the movement to redefine death, primarily as a mechanism to improve organ procurement, was predicated on and locked into place the unexamined reliance on the so-called dead-donor rule. This principle is often posited as a starting point for organ retrieval, as if its rationale were self-evident. According to this principle, a patient must be dead before his or her organs can be removed. My contention is that there is ample precedent in the law and good moral justification for removing organs from persons who are not legally dead" (172).

Thus, instead of redefining death to facilitate organ donation, Fost claims that we would be better off abandoning the dead-donor rule. He believes there are many patients who are not dead—such as anencephalics, individuals in PermVS, and others for whom planned death is the morally preferable course—whose interests (if they have any) in continued life would not be compromised by allowing them to become organ donors. Abandoning the dead-donor rule and finding more narrow justifications and legal rationales—based on principles of utility and respect for autonomy—for the removal of organs and discontinuation of life support would expand the pool of potential organ donors. In addition, "It would have the virtue of no longer claiming that we know something that is beyond our expertise or capacity to know—namely, when a person is dead. We would no longer have to ask next of kin to use or accept a word—*death*—in situations where it makes little intuitive sense" (175).

Fost is right to challenge the assumption in the biological paradigm that we know when a person is dead on the basis of objective biological considerations. This "noble lie" or fiction cannot be justified and in the long run does more harm than good. I think, however, that Fost underestimates the role of ontological considerations in our moral thinking. For example, many Catholics view suffering as having a purpose and proscribe any intentional termination of human life. They would not be receptive to moral arguments that appeal to the exercise of autonomy and lack of interest in continued life. As long as the life is a human life, they would oppose the removal of vital organs, because that would be viewed as a deliberate termination of life. This would be outside the bounds of what they consider a morally permissible exercise of autonomy. It would make a great difference in their thinking, however, if they accepted on ontological grounds, for example, that the life of an anencephalic or an individual in PermVS was not a human life or no longer the life of a person. The moral restrictions that they believe apply to persons would no longer be binding, and this would presumably allow for organ donation.[12] These ontological arguments, however, involve considerations that go beyond the narrower moral and legal principles that Fost believes would be sufficient to justify and expand the pool of potential organ donors.

In my view, the preferable course of action would be to come clean on the fact that defining death is more than a biological matter and to more honestly address the challenges posed by advances in medical technology to our understanding of who and what we are. Just as technological advances enable persons to live in ways that previously were impossible, they enable us to die in ways that were previously impossible. We should face this reality directly and not avoid the fundamental issue by some bit of practical moral reasoning that may or may not fit with our deeper metaphysical beliefs. The dead-donor rule not only may serve as a practical check to abuse, as in the Wada case, but may be a reflection of the significance of ontology to our moral thinking and our aim to get at the truth about our nature. The approach that Fost advocates ignores the deeper metaphysical and cultural dimensions of the problem.[13]

The President's Commission (1981) rejected Dworkin's approach, mainly on the grounds that multiple definitions of death would create confusion in the law and would conflict with an understanding of death as a biological fact or reality. I have already presented arguments that challenge any appeal to the "biological reality" of death, as any definition of human death depends on beliefs about human nature and personhood that go beyond biology. As to the "confusion" that would be engendered by adopting multiple definitions or allowing individuals to choose among alternatives, the commission never elaborates on why and what type of confusion would result. This objection is voiced, but it is unclear exactly what it amounts to.

One of the few writers to consider in more detail what social confusion or policy chaos might result from a more pluralistic approach to defining death is Robert Veatch, but he argues persuasively that these concerns are overblown. He notes that we already allow individual choice about withholding or withdrawing medical treatment and that this freedom has not caused abuse of patients or undue stress on health professionals, family, and public institutions, such as hospitals and courts. If anything, Veatch believes, the potential for abuse is greater in granting patients and surrogates the right to decide about withholding or withdrawing life support than it would be in granting them the right to decide on a definition of death (Veatch 1999, 149). Moreover, he considers the possibility of abuse or chaos resulting from allowing individuals to choose among alternative definitions of death in several specific contexts, such as health insurance, life insurance, inheritance, marital status, organ transplantation, succession to the presidency, and the effect on health professionals. In each of these contexts, he argues, allowing the additional freedom of choice would not create chaos and could be reasonably accommodated.

Since Veatch believes the choice of a definition of death is a "religious/philosophical/policy choice rather than a question of medical science" (156), he argues on the grounds of liberalism and democratic pluralism for inclusion of a conscience clause in the legal definition of death that would allow individual patients (or, in some cases, their next of kin) to choose, within reason, an alternative definition. Veatch notes that, although the constitutional protection of freedom of religion does not guarantee absolute freedom of religious action, the burden on the state to justify interference with religious practice is very great. The state would have to demonstrate that there would be significant social harm if people were allowed to exercise choice about the definition of death. As Veatch argues, such harm cannot be shown.

Veatch proposes that states should choose a default definition (probably, in his view, the whole-brain criterion) and then grant individuals "a limited range of discretion within the limits of reason" for conscientious objection to the default definition (177). This range would include the two other main criteria for determining death that have been proposed: (1) the irreversible loss of circulation and respiration and (2) the irreversible loss of consciousness. Individuals could exercise their choice as part of their advance directive. Unless a stronger case could be made for limiting freedom in this area, I would agree with Veatch that such a pluralistic proposal seems to be the most humane, respectful, fair, and pragmatic thing to do.

I would revise Veatch's proposal, however, to reflect what I have argued is the correct conceptual basis for accepting the various criteria for determining death: the breakdown of the psychophysical integrity of the person. Such a concept would allow for alternative religious and philosophical interpretations and acceptance of alternative criteria for determining death consistent with those interpretations. For example, the traditional notion of death as the separation of the soul from the body is consistent with this conceptual formulation. Individuals could then decide which criterion (circulatory and respiratory, whole brain, or higher-brain) is consistent with their understanding of psychophysical integrity. Those who are, like Veatch, committed to a Judeo-Christian understanding of the person as a substantial union of mind and body and think the irreversible loss of higher-brain functions would result in the destruction of this union could accept irreversible loss of higher-brain functions as a criterion of death. Others, like Shewmon and Byrne, who believe a human organism that has lost all brain functions still retains its soul or spirit and thus has not lost its psychophysical integrity could accept only the loss of circulation and respiration as a criterion for determining death. Finally, those who, like Ramsay, believe the person's psychophysical integrity would be destroyed by the loss of all brain functions but not by the loss of only higher-brain functions could accept a whole-brain criterion of death.

Notes

1. Proponents of this view include Eric Olson (1997), Fred Feldman (1992), P. F. Snowdon (1990, 1991), and Alexander Morgan Capron (1987).

2. Proponents of this view include John Locke ([1694] 1975), David Hume ([1739] 1978), Derek Parfit (1986), James Bernat (1998), and Bernat, Charles Culver, and Bernard Gert (1981, 1982a).

3. Proponents of this view include Boethius *Contra Eutychen et Nestorium* 3, Peter Strawson (1959), and David Wiggins (1980).

INTRODUCTION: THE BIOLOGICAL PARADIGM OF DEATH

1. I use the terms *higher-brain functions* and *lower-brain functions* to distinguish between those brain functions that are necessary and sufficient for consciousness, sentience, and thought and those that are not. The identification of which brain functions are necessary and sufficient is, of course, unsettled and is the focus of much current research in neurobiology. Also, there is some evidence that the common assumption in neurology that cortical structures and functions are necessary for consciousness, sentience, and thought may be mistaken. See, e.g., Shewmon (1992, 2004a) and Plum (1991).

2. Anencephaly is defined as "a severe and uniformly fatal abnormality resulting in the congenital absence of skull, scalp, and forebrain. Although some telencephalic tissue may be present, by the time of birth, there is no functional cortex but only a hemorrhagic mass of neurons and glia" (Shinnar and Arras 1989, 730). J.-M. Guérit expresses the view widely accepted in neurology that anencephaly constitutes a "pathophysiological process known to be incompatible with consciousness, irrespective of whether the brain stem is functioning or not" (Guérit 2004, 19–20). There is some debate, however, over whether the plasticity of the brain may enable some infants lacking cortical structures to have experiences that would normally be mediated by these structures in adults (Shewmon 1988, 1992, 2004a). Indeed, D. Alan Shewmon (2004a) reports three remarkable cases in which children without cortical structures exhibited conscious behavior.

Shewmon (1988) estimates that approximately 1,125 anencephalic infants are born each year in the United States. About one-half are stillborn. Of the other half, most studies report that 90 to 100 percent die in the first week. Survival beyond a few weeks has been reported in some cases (Shinnar and Arras 1989; Medical Task Force on Anencephaly 1990; Lemire, Beckwith, and Warkany 1978; Baird and Sadovnik 1984; Elwood and Elwood 1980; Peabody and Emery 1989; Pomerance and Schifrin 1987).

3. I use the term *permanent vegetative state* (PermVS) to refer to extreme cases of persistent vegetative state (PVS) in which the diagnosis of the irreversible loss of consciousness and other cognitive functions can be determined with a high degree of probability. The Multi-Society Task Force on PVS states that "a permanent vegetative state . . . means an irreversible state, which like all clinical diagnoses in medicine, is based on probabilities, not absolutes. A patient in a persistent vegetative state becomes permanently vegetative when the diagnosis of irreversibility can be established with a high degree of clinical certainty—that is when the chance that the patient will regain consciousness is exceedingly small" (Multi-Society Task Force 1994, 1501). Guérit (1994, 1995) identifies such cases pathophysiologically by their absence of all primary components of cortical evoked potentials (EPs). In a later publication he explains:

> We know that, for metabolic reasons, the sensitivity to anoxia of the primary sensory cortices is intermediate between that of association cortex and brain stem (Plum and Posner 1980, 87–151). This implies that brain anoxia sufficient to destroy the primary cortex should be sufficient to destroy all association cortex, irrespective of brain stem status. This irreversible situation is incompatible with any consciousness . . . Significantly, this situation can be reliably identified at the patient's bedside with multimodality or, more specifically, somatosensory EPs, which show the absence of any cortical components [what we labeled as post-anoxic Grade 4 in our EP classification (Guérit et al. 1993)]. One major advantage of this approach is that Grade 4 somatosensory EPs constitute a pattern clearly distinct from all others, eliminating any "slippery slope." (Guérit 2004, 20, bracketed comment in original; reference to Guérit et al. 1993 in footnote in original)

There is some debate, however, over whether we can know that individuals in PVS lack consciousness, temporarily or irreversibly. See Howsepian (1994, 1996), Borthwick (1996), Shewmon (2004a), and Laureys et al. (2004). My use of the term *PermVS* stipulates an irreversible loss of consciousness, and thus most of my arguments regarding such individuals can be considered independently of the empirical issue of which individuals are in this state.

4. Others who have recognized that the matter of defining death goes beyond biological considerations and involves consideration of the nature of personhood or humanity include George Agich (1976), H. Tristram Engelhardt, Jr. (1978), Jeff McMahan (1995, 2002), James Smith (1982), and Robert Veatch (1972, 1976, 1993).

5. If death is not a type of ceasing to exist, then it is unclear what *would* count as a type of ceasing to exist. For a challenge to the claim that a person's death does not entail the person's ceasing to exist, see Fred Feldman (1992, ch. 6).

6. By *essential*, I follow Aristotle's understanding of an essential property as a property that is necessary for something to exist as the kind of thing that it is. Its loss would therefore entail the ceasing to exist of that kind of thing (Aristotle *Metaphysics* 7). This view does not entail understanding every aspect or characteristic of a person in more than purely biological terms. Persons undergo a host of biological activity that can be explained and predicted in purely bi-

ological terms. My claim is that the issue of when the life of a human being or person ends, as when it begins, cannot be understood in purely biological terms. This is because persons and human beings are not simply biological beings.

CHAPTER 1. ESTABLISHMENT OF THE BIOLOGICAL PARADIGM

1. For helpful discussions of the history of the development of the concept and criteria of "brain death," see David Lamb (1990, 31–36), Robert Veatch (1978, 19–21), Martin S. Pernick (1999), and Calixto Machado (in press).

2. For the specific state statutes, regulations, and case law that have recognized the criteria for determining death in the Uniform Determination of Death Act, see Charles M. Kester (1994, nn. 44–46).

3. Section 26:6A-5 of the New Jersey Declaration of Death Act reads: "Death not declared in violation of individual's religious beliefs. The death of an individual shall not be declared upon the basis of neurological criteria pursuant to sections 3 and 4 of this act when the licensed physician authorized to declare death, has reason to believe, on the basis of information in the individual's available medical records, or information provided by a member of the individual's family or any other person knowledgeable about the individual's personal religious beliefs that such a declaration would violate the personal religious beliefs of the individual. In these cases, death shall be declared, and the time of death fixed, solely upon the basis of cardio-respiratory criteria pursuant to section 2 of this act, L.1991, c90, s5" (www.braindeath.org/law/newjersey/htm). See also Orlick (1991). For an interesting commentary on this "conscience clause," see Veatch (1999).

4. This is perhaps no surprise, as Alexander Capron served as the executive director of the President's Commission.

5. For persuasive critiques of the claim that acceptance of a neurological criterion for determining death does not introduce a new meaning or concept of death, see Karen Gervais (1986, 18–44) and Robert M. Veatch (1993).

6. In this view, what it means for the anencephalic to come into existence and die is tied to conceptions of the kind of being the anencephalic is—a human being, humanoid, or some other kind. These conditions differ from those for persons. For an interesting objection to the whole-brain criterion of death based on consideration of what it means for an early fetus to die, see Ingmar Persson (2002).

7. George Agich (1976), Christopher Pallis (1983), David Lamb (1985), and Tom Russell (2000) also note the difficulty of trying to propose criteria without having a clear idea what the criteria are for. Russell asserts, "Criteria for death can have meaning only if they can be shown to be logically derived from the appropriate concept of death . . . It is meaningless to use 'free-floating criteria' that are not derived from a clearly determined concept of death" (Russell 2000, 60). While I agree with Russell that criteria cannot be "free floating" and need to be logically linked to a concept of death, it is unclear how "clearly determined" the concept must be. For example, one reason why Lamb rejects a consciousness-related definition of death is that he thinks such a concept cannot be clearly determined. Hans Jonas (1974), however, urges us to admit some "vagueness" in our concept or definition of death, because he believes there

is vagueness in our concept of the nature of a human being. I agree with Jonas. I believe our concepts of *human being* and *person* are inherently vague in the sense that they are never completely determined but are open-ended projects. These concepts are determined by biological, metaphysical, moral, and cultural factors. Accordingly, the vagueness in these concepts forces us to accept a certain vagueness in any concepts of the coming into existence and ceasing to exist (death) of these beings. The nature of human beings or persons is not something that is discovered. Our concepts of human being and person are thus not timelessly fixed in the sense that natural kind terms may be fixed. (See chapter 2, n. 3, for more on natural kind.)

8. In Polish there are two separate words for death—one used for animals and the other for persons. On the variety of different uses of the term across cultures and languages, see Shewmon and Shewmon (2004).

CHAPTER 2. DEFINING DEATH

1. I thank Robert Taylor for his help in constructing this hypothetical case.

2. The issue of whether we should abandon the common assumption that death is irreversible has been addressed in the recent literature, especially in the context of non-heart-beating organ donation. See, e.g., Cole (1992, 1993), Lamb (1992), Lynn (1993), Tomlinson (1993), and Bartlett (1995). I also discuss this issue elsewhere (Lizza 2005).

3. The view of "natural kind" appealed to is that developed by Hilary Putnam (1970), Saul Kripke (1972), and David Wiggins (1980) and can be traced back to Leibniz and Aristotle. Paraphrasing Wiggins (1980, 77–86, 169–75), the determination of a natural kind depends on the existence of lawlike principles that collect together the actual extension of the kind around an arbitrarily good specimen of it and that determine the characteristic activity, development, and history of members of this extension.

4. For the distinction between substance and phased sortals and further discussion of these notions, see Wiggins (1980, 24–27, 59, 64) and my discussion in chapter 7.

CHAPTER 3. CONCEPTS OF PERSON

1. I discuss the concept of potentiality in more detail in chapter 6.

2. For such an open-ended concept of person, see Wiggins (1980, ch. 6).

3. For an earlier account of these distinct senses of *person* and how they can be used in an analysis of dissociative personality disorder, see Lizza (1993a). In this earlier work, I called the second meaning of person an "appearance meaning" and its third meaning, a "reality meaning." Here I refer to the second meaning of person as a "qualitative meaning" and the third meaning as a "substantive meaning." These latter terms are more descriptive of the semantic distinctions that I wish to draw.

4. I thank Christopher Bryant for the specific example of the sign in an elevator.

5. For a critical discussion of this particular point, see Rosenberg (1983, ch. 4).

6. In the preface to his book *The Human Animal* (1997), Olson admits that it is hard to find anyone in the history of Western philosophy who identifies the person with the human organism regardless of whether that organism has the potential or capacity for psychological states.

7. Examples are anencephalics, individuals in PermVS, and the artificially sustained, whole-brain dead. I shall argue for this view in more detail in my discussion in chapter 6 of the "species meaning" sense of personhood and the views of Seifert and Shewmon.

8. If we were to apply the basic metaphysical distinction between a substance and property/mode, the "species meaning" of person would fall under the category of substance because it treats the person as a substantive entity (i.e., human organism) rather than a mode of an entity. Here, however (to reiterate), I am using "substantive meaning" to refer to views that treat persons as substantive entities with essentially the potential or capacity for consciousness and other mental functions.

9. Robert Veatch, personal communication, June 4, 1994, Essex House, New York.

10. Macklin does not explicitly say that the disagreement over personhood is "fundamental," but her conclusion that no further progress can be made through further investigation of the alternative concepts of personhood seems to imply as much. Otherwise, what other reason would there be for such a claim?

11. In chapter 7, I critique Derek Parfit's claim that personal survival rather than personal identity is what matters to us, on the grounds that Parfit's thought experiments distort our understanding of what matters precisely because they sunder persons from their social-cultural-historical context.

CHAPTER 4. PERSONS AS SUBSTANCES

1. See, e.g., Thomas Aquinas *Summa Theologiae* 1.75–89, Gilson (1940, 189–208; 1956, 187–222), and Donceel (1970).

2. For further defense of a substantive view of persons, although not the specific version that I defend in this work, see Lowe (1989, 1991a, 1991b) and Honnefelder (1996).

3. I accept the claim that identity is absolute. See Wiggins (1980, ch. 1) for a strong defense of the view.

4. Strawson is uncertain whether anyone has actually held this view. He does suggest that it may been held at one time by Wittgenstein and Schlick. I do not see why the view cannot be attributed to Hume. When Hume looked inside himself to see who the owner or subject of his experiences was, he couldn't find one. He claimed to be aware of particular experiences, but of no "I" or self. He concluded that there is no "I" over and above the experiences and thus the "I" is nothing but a bundle of experiences related to each other in certain ways.

5. While E. J. Lowe (1991a, 90–95) correctly interprets Wiggins as advocating a substantive view of persons, Lowe seems to miss Wiggins's qualification that *person* is "similar" or "akin" to a natural kind concept, rather than being a natural kind concept. Lowe misinterprets Wiggins as holding that persons *are* a natural, biological kind.

6. Concepts are "sortally concordant" if they agree on the persistence conditions that they ascribe to an individual lying within their extension. See Wiggins (1980, 65; 204–5, n. 2.10).

7. Wiggins cites Davidson ([1970] 2001). The reference to Moore is presumably to *Principia Ethica* ([1903] 1993).

8. See Wiggins's discussion (1980, 23–27) of purported type-(3) cases of relative identity.

CHAPTER 5. THE CONSTITUTIVE VIEW OF PERSONS

1. As far as I am aware, the first author to propose that persons may be constituted by but not identical to bodies was Sidney Shoemaker (Shoemaker and Swinburne 1984, 113–14).

2. A most significant aspect of Baker's theory is her treatment of constitution as a "unity relation" (i.e., when *x* constitutes *y*, there are not two things that happen to spatiotemporally coincide but a single thing, *y* as constituted by *x*) (Baker 2000, 46). This leads to a distinction between how things can have properties derivatively and nonderivatively (cf. Persson 1999), a distinction that enables Baker (2000, 191–212) to fend off some of the more forceful objections from the animalist camp leveled by Olson (1997) and Snowdon (1990). For her further defense of the constitutive view, see Baker (1999, 2002).

3. On this sense of nomological grounding or *de re* necessity involved with natural kinds, see also Putnam (1970, 1975) and Kripke (1972).

4. Prince did not believe every "sick" self is an "artificial" self. Many people, for example, exhibit neurasthenia and aboulia, but that does not make them "artificial." Several factors led Prince to the diagnosis of the artificial status of the various personalities in the Beauchamp case: his observation of what may be a unique combination of symptoms exhibited by multiple personalities, his physical and psychological testing of the personalities, his consideration of their causal history, and a comparison of the phenomena exhibited by the multiple personalities with other dissociative states. For further discussion of my view of dissociative personality disorder, see Lizza (1993a).

5. E. J. Lowe (1989) goes a step further by conceiving of immaterial persons and rejecting the constitutive view for this reason. The conceivability of a person continuing to exist in an immaterial substance leads him to think that having a body is not essential to a person.

6. On this sense of *de re* necessity, see Wiggins (1974; 1976; 1980, ch. 4), Kirwan (1970–71), and Burge (1977).

7. Cf. Shoemaker (1970, 270).

8. Leibniz seems to have recognized how our identity is determined by how others regard us when he considers the possibility of brain zap and observes, "if I forgot my whole past and needed to have myself taught all over again, even my name and how to read and write, I could still learn from others about my life during my preceding state; and similarly, I would have retained my rights without having to be divided into persons and made to inherit from myself" (Leibniz [1690] 1981, paras. 236–37).

9. In an earlier work (Lizza 1993a), I criticized Wilkes's claim that moral and social considerations explain why we do not treat cases of dissociative personality disorder as bona fide cases of more than one person in a single body. I now believe these factors do play a role, in addition to the role played by theoretical assumptions in psychology about persons as or as akin to natural kinds.

CHAPTER 6. PERSONS AS HUMAN ORGANISMS

1. In support of his interpretation of Wiggins's view, Christopher Gill cites Wiggins (1987, 56, 66–67). See also Wiggins (1980, ch. 6).

2. Gill notes at this point that "from our experience of human-beings-viewed-as-persons, we are able to piece out the necessary incompleteness of any philosophical definition of the 'person,' such as Locke's." Gill refers to Wiggins (1987, 68–69). The quoted material in Gill's next paragraph is from Wiggins (1987, 71).

3. See also Thomson (1987).

4. Holmes Rolston (1982) argues for a "naturalistic principle" that involves respect for biological (objective) life devoid of all subjective experience. For a critique of Rolston's view, see Freer (1984).

5. Among "philosophers in the Western tradition" I include major figures from Plato to de Beauvoir. While philosophers in the tradition disagree about what they take to be sufficient for personhood, there is a great deal of consensus that, minimally, the potential for consciousness is required. Contemporary philosophers, such as Olson, Feldman, and Snowdon, are the exception. Olson (1997) makes this observation in the first chapter of *The Human Animal*.

6. The view that any human being is a person (i.e., has the full moral status that we normally accord to human beings or persons) has also figured prominently in the abortion debate, notably in the writings of John Noonan and R. E. Joyce. Even in their most conservative arguments against abortion, however, *person* is still defined as a being with the "potential" or "capacity" for psychological functions. Joyce (1998, 200) defines *person* as "a whole individual being which has the natural potential to know, love, desire, and relate to self and others in a self-reflective way." While this definition may support the claim that normal human fetuses are persons, it does not support the claim that anencephalics or individuals in PermVS are persons. Because these individuals lack the physiological basis for the "potential to know, love, desire," they cannot be persons.

Noonan (1968, 134) holds that "everyone is human who is conceived of human beings." On its face, this criterion for human beings or persons seems to admit anencephalics and individuals in PermVS into the class of human beings or persons. If we look closer at Noonan's argument for adopting this criterion, however, we see that it assumes that any product of human conception would have, as he puts it, "the capacity for rational thought" (135). Because this assumption underlies his criterion of humanity or personhood, the criterion is inconsistent with the claim that individuals lacking the potential or capacity for psychological functions, including rationality, are persons.

7. Strictly speaking, we would have to say that the anencephalic never existed as a person, rather than that the anencephalic person had "died."

8. Plato's view in the *Phaedo* is clearly dualistic and influenced by the Pythagorean doctrine that immaterial souls are periodically reincarnated in material bodies.

9. In this context, Shewmon (1985, 53) cites the following from Aquinas's *Summa Theologiae* 1.76.5.2: "A body is not necessary to the intellectual soul by reason of its intellectual operation considered as such, but because of the sensitive power, which requires an organ harmoniously tempered. Therefore the intellectual soul had to be united to such a body, and not to a simple element." Shewmon concludes, "St. Thomas is therefore almost as explicit as he could be, within the context of the medical knowledge of his day, in suggesting that respiratory arrest results in death, not because respiration *per se* is of the essence of life, but because it leads to the necrosis of the cerebral hemispheres . . . At the time of St. Thomas, medical

men believed that the organ of the cogitative sense was one of the ventricles in the middle of the head" (Shewmon 1985, 53–54).

10. Shewmon writes, "In the case of higher forms of life, such as animals and man, the accidental changes immediately responsible for death are usually also changes which attack the unifying principle at the vegetative level: i.e., irreversible loss of integrity of the cells throughout the body. As the soul quits the body, the body becomes a great mixture of chemicals. However, suppose the accidental changes attacked the essence of the organism at a level higher than vegetative. There is no a priori reason to exclude the possibility of a higher level soul being superseded by a lower level soul, rather than by a mixture of inanimate forms" (Shewmon 1985, 41).

11. Aristotle explains that "the seed is not yet potentially a man; for it must be deposited in something other than itself and undergo a change" (*Metaphysics* 9.7.1049a14–15, trans. Ross).

12. I owe this example to Allan Back.

13. Aquinas held that the ensoulment of ordinary human beings took place over time, as the matter had to be developed in order to be ensouled; if the ensoulment were to take place without properly disposed matter, the ensoulment would be miraculous. As William Wallace points out, Aquinas held that "Christ's conception, unlike that of other humans, should not have to await the complete formation of his natural flesh. On this account Christ was conceived instantly by the divine power of the Holy Spirit, and thus in miraculous fashion (*In 3 Sent.*, d.3, q.5,a,2)" (Wallace 1995, 395). See also Donceel (1970, 79ff.)

14. Part of the justification for this view comes from acceptance of David Wiggins's view (indebted to Putnam and more distantly to Leibniz and Aristotle) that natural kinds are delineated by activities that members of the kind characteristically have (Wiggins 1980, ch. 6). When a member of a kind loses activity that is deemed essential for membership in that kind, we should conclude that the member has died or ceased to exist. Thus, if human beings and persons have, as Wiggins suggests, a "neo-Lockean" principle of individuation and identity grounded in psychological activity and they lose their capacity for psychological activity, then a substantial change in kind has taken place. Thus, I would question the assumption that artificially sustained, brain-dead or decapitated human bodies are members of the human species. This is also why I think Shewmon got it right in his earlier paper when he treated such beings as humanoid but not human or members of the human species. In my view, technology has made it possible to change one kind of living thing into another kind of living thing and has thereby made it possible for us to die in ways that were previously impossible. Note also that the determination of what kinds of things there are is not independent of interests and values. Thus, the ethical considerations advanced for the relevance of realistic potentials, rather than potentials that are remote or independent of material conditions, would also argue in favor of treating the loss of all brain functions as a substantial change in the human organism.

15. For a discussion of how a concept of realistic potentiality applies in the abortion context with respect to evaluating the moral significance of the potentialities of the conceptus at various developmental stages, see Langerak (1979).

16. The Multi-Society Task Force on PVS stated that "a permanent vegetative state . . . means an irreversible state, which like all clinical diagnoses in medicine is based on probabilities, not absolutes. A patient in a persistent vegetative state becomes permanently vegetative when the diagnosis of irreversibility can be established with a high degree of clinical cer-

tainty—that is when the chance that the patient will regain consciousness is exceedingly small." In this context, the task force distinguishes a realistic, practical sense of "irreversibility" or "lack of potential for consciousness" from the more theoretical, "promiscuous" sense of potentiality (Multi-Society Task Force 1994, 1501).

17. The bishop who read from the report indicated that it was not a public document. I have been unable to obtain the report.

18. See, e.g., Eberl (2005) for a different interpretation of Aquinas's understanding of death. Eberl, however, never critically addresses Wallace's interpretation. In addition, although Eberl notes that Shewmon now holds that the brain is not crucial for the integration of the human organism, he fails to explain why he does not follow Shewmon in rejecting the neurological criteria for death.

CHAPTER 7. PERSONS AS QUALITIES OR PHASES OF HUMAN ORGANISMS

1. For more on the distinction between a phased predicate (phased sortal concept) and substance predicate (substance sortal concept), see David Wiggins (1980, ch. 1).

2. See Wiggins (1980, 23–24) for a discussion of the purported case of relative identity, involving the phase sortal "boy": "John Doe, the boy whom they thought a dunce at school, is the *same human being* as Sir John Doe, the Lord Mayor of London, but not the *same boy* (for the Lord Mayor is not a boy)."

3. This intuition is shared by those who *identify* persons with human organisms, because they believe it is the persistence of a substance or entity (i.e., the human organism) and not some relation between psychological states or events that accounts for what makes the someone the same person over time. On the species view, personal identity consists of bodily continuity, not psychological continuity.

4. Cf. Wiggins's account of *C, discussed in chapter 5.

5. Michael Lockwood notes that one might respond to this objection to the memory criterion by the counterfactual supposition that, if we woke the person, the person would be able to report memories. I do not think this response would work, because there would still be unconscious states of the person that would not be linked. If our unconscious is a part of who we are, then it should be incorporated into any adequate criterion of personal identity. It is hard to see how memory could do this.

6. This passage from Leibniz is also quoted by Allison (1966).

7. Parfit uses the expression "what matters" to talk about what is important or of primary concern to us about persons and identity. For example, when he writes, "Personal identity is not what matters. What fundamentally matters is Relation R [psychological continuity] with any cause," I interpret him to mean that Relation R is all that matters to us in terms of rational, egoistic concern (Parfit 1986, 217; cf. McMahan 2002, 41–43).

8. In *Reasons and Persons* (1986), Parfit claimed that personal identity and reality, in general, could be described *impersonally* (i.e., without making reference to persons). More recently (Parfit 1999, 254), he says this was a mistake. In his later work, he retains the concept of *person* as a phase of the human organism, but thus continues to reject the idea that *person* as a substantive entity is necessary for any adequate theory of reality.

9. In his later work, Parfit (1999, 218) says that the kind of reductionism he espouses holds that "we are distinct from our bodies and brains, though we are not, in relation to them, separately existing entities. This we can call Constitutive Reductionism." He accepts the distinction between persons and their bodies or brains because he accepts that they have different persistence conditions. Unlike Shoemaker, Baker, and myself, Parfit does not think we are essentially persons. He thinks we are essentially human beings and treats the concept *person* as a phased sortal. Parfit also seems to want to distinguish his view from the species view or animalism that identifies the person with the human being. He calls this view "hyperreductionism" (Parfit 1999, 219). His view of a constitutive relation between the person and human body (organism) thus differs from that relation as understood by Baker and Shoemaker, because it does not treat the concept *person* as a primitive concept or substance sortal. Also, as I show later in the chapter, Parfit seems to reject Baker's claims (2000, 41) that "it is only in certain circumstances . . . that one thing constitutes another" and that persons, along with other things that are constituted (e.g., works of art), have essential relational properties.

10. In Baker's view, this dependency is understood in terms of "global supervenience" and "constitution."

11. Parfit (1999) responds at length to these objections. To discuss and respond to his response would take another book. I will just comment that, as in *Reasons and Persons*, Parfit continues to separate the metaphysical and moral issues about persons in a way that I would not. This will be evident in the discussion later in this chapter of what I find to be the second main difficulty with Parfit's view.

12. The passage from McGinn is also cited by Maslin (2001, 271, n. 6). For a further challenge to the notion of quasi-memory, see Wiggins (2001, ch. 7).

13. The question may be raised about whether someone would cease to be a person *simply* because he was no longer regarded as one by the society to which he happened to belong (e.g., a Jew under Nazi persecution). The answer is no. Because *person* is a metaphysical and moral concept in addition to a cultural one, resources from our moral and metaphysical theories could be invoked to counter the claim (e.g., there was no moral justification for the Nazis' treatment of Jews as nonpersons).

14. This argument was originally presented elsewhere (Lizza 1991). For a criticism of Parfit along similar lines, see S. White (1989).

15. I thank Michael Griffith for his comments on an earlier version of this argument that I presented at the 1996 Pacific Division Meeting of the American Philosophical Association. The elaboration on Parfit's thought experiment of the Combined Spectrum to frame the issue of whether extrinsic factors would influence one's judgments about personal identity is Griffith's. Griffith, however, used the thought experiment—unsuccessfully, in my view—to show that extrinsic factors would *not* matter to our judgments about personal identity.

16. For more developed psychological theories of how a person's identity over time is dependent on self-conceptions that are in turn dependent on social factors of recognition and reinforcement, see, e.g., Erikson (1956) and Harré (1984).

17. If Parfit were to adopt his more recent (1999) terminology of "Constitutive Reductionism," the analogy of persons to nations would seem awkward. Because Parfit says that he understands persons as phases of human organisms, the analogy would seem to entail a nation

being a phase of its citizens, living together in certain ways on its territory. Prima facie, this strikes me as an odd thing to say.

18. This discussion of Tännsjö's work refers to his "Morality and personal identity," in *Spinning Ideas: Electronic Essays Dedicated to Peter Gardenfors on His Fiftieth Birthday* (www.lucs.lu.se/spinning/categories/moral/Tannsjo/index/html).

CHAPTER 8. PUBLIC POLICY AND THE DEFINITION OF DEATH

1. See Brock (1987) for his broader reflections on this issue.

2. For a good discussion of the "dead donor" rule, see Arnold and Youngner (1995).

3. This comparison was also pointed out by Youngner and Bartlett (1983, 254). Shewmon clarifies the significance of the comparison in the following way:

> If the brain is uniquely responsible for the organism's biological unity, so that in the absence of the brain's coordinating activity the organism becomes a mere disunited collection of organs and tissues, such somatic "dis-integration" should be just the same regardless whether the absence of brain-coordination is due to absence of a brain or merely to functional disconnection from the brain. Thus, various brain disconnection syndromes might provide important insights into the nature of BD [brain death]. If the somatic physiologies are indeed similar, if not identical, as theoretically they should be, then however terms such as "organism as a whole" might be operationally defined, if they apply or do not apply to brain disconnection, they must equally apply or not apply to BD. The "central-integrator-of-the-body" rationale of BD can therefore be tested by examining the vital status of the brain-disconnected bodies, so long as the somatic physiology of the two conditions is indeed equivalent. (Shewmon 2004b, 24)

4. In a recent study, Laureys et al. (2004, 236) conclude that "at present, the potential for recovery of awareness from the VS [vegetative state] cannot be predicted reliably by any clinical or neurodiagnostic test."

5. See, e.g., Ludwig Wittgenstein's "beetle in the box" argument (1953, sect. 293).

6. For an excellent account of how Wittgenstein's theory of meaning applies in this context, see Gillett (1990).

7. P. F. Strawson's view has to be defended to show that it does not entail commitment to some form of logical or ontological behaviorism, as, for example, Graham (1993, 39–40) and G. Strawson (1994, 223–24) have charged. Also, A. J. Ayer (1963, 105–6) argued that Strawson's view begs the question by assuming that other people are conscious, which is the very point at issue. These criticisms are pointed out by Maslin (2001, ch. 8).

8. An obvious target for Shewmon's question would be the American Academy of Neurology, when, in its *amicus curiae* brief submitted in *Brophy v. New England*, it stated unequivocally, "No conscious experience of pain and suffering is possible without the integrated functioning of the brainstem and cerebral cortex. Pain and suffering are attributes of consciousness, and PVS [persistent vegetative state] patients like Brophy do not experience them. Noxious stimuli may activate peripherally located nerves, but only a brain with the capacity

for consciousness can translate that neural activity into an experience. That part of Brophy's brain is forever lost" (398 Mass. 417 N.E.2d 626 [1986]).

9. Andrews reaches the same conclusion: "Accurate diagnosis is possible but requires the skill of a multidisciplinary team experienced in the management of people with complex disabilities . . . a quarter of those diagnosed as vegetative by the referring team remained vegetative and were almost certainly, from our experience, likely to remain so. These findings are therefore not an argument against the withdrawal of artificial nutrition and hydration but do emphasize the importance of accurate diagnosis of the vegetative state being made after expert assessment and provision of a rehabilitation programme by a very experienced team" (Andrews 1996, 13–16).

10. Dworkin gives examples from different areas of law in which special definitions of death have already been adopted:

> Numerous property and wealth transmission issues raise death questions: When may an estate be probated? When may property of a testate or intestate decedent be distributed? When does a life estate end? When does property pass to a surviving joint tenant? When do life insurance benefits become payable and health insurance benefits cease to accrue? When may property escheat? When do agents, conservators, attorneys and trustees lose their authority to act, and when do banks become liable for admitting persons to safe deposit boxes and paying money out of accounts? When is an estate tax due? When is a gift within three years of death so that it may be said to be in contemplation of death? . . . [What determines whether] a person who remarries is a bigamist and whether the remarriage is valid? (Dworkin 1973, 631)

11. Lock refers to Bai (1970, 41) in support of her interpretation.

12. This was the reasoning for why the group of Catholic bioethicists cited in chapter 6 did not oppose organ donation from anencephalic infants.

13. Fost recognizes that declaring death at a certain point in time plays an important role in the ritual of saying good-bye and grieving for a loved one. He also states, however, "it is helpful and desirable to select a point in time where it is appropriate to say, 'He is dead,' not because it is true, or because we are expert on such questions, or because it facilitates organ retrieval, but because it is helpful" (Fost 1999, 175). This pragmatic rationale for deciding when someone is dead is too limited. It ignores the relevance of ontology to our moral thinking.

References

Ad Hoc Committee of the Harvard Medical School to Examine the Definition of Brain Death. 1968. A definition of irreversible coma. *Journal of the American Medical Association* 205:337–340.

Agich, G. J. 1976. The concepts of death and embodiment. *Ethics in Science and Medicine* 3:95–105.

Allison, H. 1966. Locke's theory of personal identity: A re-examination. *Journal of the History of Ideas* 27:41–58.

American Academy of Neurology. 1989. Position statement of the American Academy of Neurology on certain aspects of the care and management of the persistent vegetative state patient. *Neurology* 39:125–126.

Andrews, K., Murphy, L., Munday, R., and Littlewood, C. 1996. Misdiagnosis of the vegetative state: A retrospective study in a rehabilitation unit. *British Medical Journal* 313:13–16.

Annis, D. B. 1984. Abortion and the potentiality principle. *Southern Journal of Philosophy* 22:155-163.

Anstötz, A. 1993. Should a brain-dead pregnant woman carry her child to full term? The case of the "Erlanger baby." *Bioethics* 7:340–350.

Arnold, R. M., and Youngner, S. J. 1995. The dead donor rule: Should we stretch it, bend it, or abandon it? In R. M. Arnold, S. J. Youngner, R. Schapiro, and C. M. Spicer (eds.), *Procuring Organs for Transplant.* Baltimore: Johns Hopkins University Press.

Arnold, R. M., Youngner, S. J., Schapiro, R., and Spicer, C. M., eds. 1995. *Procuring Organs for Transplant.* Baltimore: Johns Hopkins University Press.

Ayer, A. J. 1963. *The Concept of a Person.* London: Macmillan.

Bai, K. 1970. Contemporary problems of medical law in Japan: Parts I and II. *Annals of the Institute of Social Science* 11:17–54.

Baird, P. A., and Sadovnik, A. D. 1984. Survival in infants with anencephaly. *Clinical Pediatrics* 23:268–271.

Baker, L. R. 1999. What am I? *Philosophy and Phenomenological Research* 59:151–159.

——. 2000. *Persons and Bodies.* Cambridge: Cambridge University Press.

——. 2002. The ontological status of persons. *Philosophy and Phenomenological Research* 65:370–388.

Bartlett, E. T. 1995. Differences between death and dying. *Journal of Medical Ethics* 21:270–276.

Beauchamp, T. L., and Perlin, S., eds. 1978. *Ethical Issues in Death and Dying*. Englewood Cliffs, NJ: Prentice-Hall.

Becker, L. 1975. Human being: The boundaries of the concept. *Philosophy and Public Affairs* 4:335–359.

Bennett, J. 1966. *Kant's Analytic*. Cambridge: Cambridge University Press.

Bernat, J. L. 1998. A defense of the whole-brain concept of death. *Hastings Center Report* 28(2):14–23.

———. 1999. Reply to J. Lizza (letter to the editor). *Hastings Center Report* 29(1):5.

———. 2002. The biophilosophical basis of whole-brain death. *Social Philosophy and Policy* 19:324–342.

Bernat, J. L., Culver, C., and Gert, B. 1981. On the definition and criterion of death. *Annals of Internal Medicine* 94:389–394.

———. 1982a. Defining death in theory and practice. *Hastings Center Report* 12(1):5–8.

———. 1982b. Reply to Robert Veatch's letter to the editor. *Hastings Center Report* 12(6):45.

Bernstein, I., Watson, M., Simmons, G. M., Catalano, M., Davis, G., and Collins, R. 1989. Maternal brain death and prolonged fetal survival. *Obstetrics and Gynecology* 74:434–437.

Blackburn, S. 1987. Has Kant refuted Parfit? In J. Dancy (ed.), *Reading Parfit*. Malden, MA: Blackwell.

Block, N. 1978. Troubles with functionalism. In C. W. Savage (ed.), *Perception and Cognition: Issues in the Foundation of Psychology* (Minnesota Studies in the Philosophy of Science, vol. 9). Minneapolis: University of Minnesota Press.

———. 1980. Are absent qualia impossible? *Philosophical Review* 89:257–274.

Block, N., and Fodor, J. 1972. What psychological states are not. *Philosophical Review* 81:159–181.

Borgman, A. 1984. *Technology and the Character of Contemporary Life*. Chicago: University of Chicago Press.

Borthwick, C. 1996. The permanent vegetative state: Ethical crux, medical fiction? *Issues in Law and Medicine* 12:167–185.

Brennan, S., and Delgado, R. 1981. Death: Multiple standards or a single standard? *Southern California Law Review* 54:1323–1355.

Brock, D. 1987. Truth or consequences: The role of philosophers in policymaking. *Ethics* 97:786–791.

———. 1999. The role of the public in public policy on the definition of death. In S. J. Youngner, R. M. Arnold, and R. Schapiro (eds.), *The Definition of Death: Contemporary Controversies*. Baltimore: Johns Hopkins University Press.

Brody, B. 1999. How much of the brain must be dead? In S. J. Youngner, R. M. Arnold, and R. Schapiro (eds.), *The Definition of Death: Contemporary Controversies*. Baltimore: Johns Hopkins University Press.

Burge, T. 1975. Mass terms, count nouns and change. *Synthese* 31:459–478.

———. 1977. Belief *de re*. *Journal of Philosophy* 74:338–362.

———. [1979] 1991. Individualism and the mental. Repr. in D. Rosenthal (ed.), *The Nature of Mind*. Oxford: Oxford University Press.

———. 1988. Individualism and self-knowledge. *Journal of Philosophy* 85:649–663.

Burt, R. A. 1999. Where do we go from here? In S. J. Youngner, R. M. Arnold, and R. Schapiro (eds.), *The Definition of Death: Contemporary Controversies*. Baltimore: Johns Hopkins University Press.

Butler, J. [1736] 1975. *The Analogy of Religion*, first appendix. Repr. in J. Perry (ed.), *Personal Identity*. Berkeley: University of California Press.

Byrne, P. A., O'Reilly, S., Quay, P., and Salsich, P. W., Jr. [1982/83] 2000. Brain death—The patient, the physician, and society. *Gonzaga Law Review* 18(3). Repr. in M. Potts, P. A. Byrne, and R. G. Nilges (eds.), *Beyond Brain Death: The Case against Brain Based Criteria for Human Death*. Dordrecht: Kluwer.

Callahan, D. 1988. The "beginning" of human life. In M. F. Goodman (ed.), *What Is a Person?* Clifton, NJ: Humana Press.

Capron, A. M. 1987. Anencephalic donors: Separate the dead from the dying. *Hastings Center Report* 17(1):5–9.

———. 1999. The bifurcated legal standard for determining death: Does it work? In S. J. Youngner, R. M. Arnold, and R. Schapiro (eds.), *The Definition of Death: Contemporary Controversies*. Baltimore: Johns Hopkins University Press.

Capron, A., and Kass, L. 1972. A statutory definition of the standards for determining human death: An appraisal and a proposal. *University of Pennsylvania Law Review* 121:87–118.

Capron, A., and Lynn, J. 1982. Reply to J. Smith's letter to the editor. *Hastings Center Report* 12(6):46.

Castañeda, H.-N. 1966. "He": A study in the logic of self-consciousness. *Ratio* 8:130–157.

Charo, R. A. 1999. Dusk, dawn, and defining death: Legal classifications and biological consequences. In S. J. Youngner, R. M. Arnold, and R. Schapiro (eds.), *The Definition of Death: Contemporary Controversies*. Baltimore: Johns Hopkins University Press.

Childs, N. L., Mercer, W. N., and Childs, H. W. 1993. Accuracy of diagnosis of persistent vegetative state. *Neurology* 43:1465–1467.

Cole, D. J. 1992. The reversibility of death. *Journal of Medical Ethics* 18:26–30.

———. 1993. Statutory definitions and the management of terminally ill patients who may become organ donors after death. *Kennedy Institute of Ethics Journal* 3:145–155.

Conee, E. 1985. The possibility of absent qualia. *Philosophical Review* 94:345–366.

Covey, E. 1991. Physical possibility and potentiality in ethics. *American Philosophical Quarterly* 28:237–244.

Cranford, R. 1988. The persistent vegetative state: The medical reality (getting the facts straight). *Hastings Center Report* 18(1):27–32.

Culver, C., and Gert, B. 1982. *Philosophy in Medicine: Conceptual and Ethical Issues in Medicine and Psychiatry*. New York: Oxford University Press.

Davidson, D. [1970] 2001. Mental events. In L. Foster and J. W. Swanson (eds.), *Experience and Theory*. London: Duckworth. Repr. in D. Davidson, *Essays on Actions and Events*. Oxford: Clarendon Press.

Descartes, R. [1641] 1986. *Meditations on First Philosophy*, trans. J. Cottingham. Cambridge: Cambridge University Press.

Donceel, J. F. 1970. Immediate animation and delayed hominization. *Theological Studies* 31:76–105.

Downie, J. 1990. Brain death and brain life: Rethinking the connection. *Bioethics* 4:216–226.

Dworkin, R. B. 1973. Death in context. *Indiana Law Journal* 48:623–639.

Eberl, J. T. 2005. A Thomistic understanding of human death. *Bioethics* 19:29–48.

Elwood, J. M., and Elwood, J. H. 1980. *Epidemiology of Anencephalics and Spina Bifida.* Oxford: Oxford University Press.

Emanuel, L. 1995. Re-examining death: The asymptotic model and a bounded zone definition. *Hastings Center Report* 25(4):27–35.

Engelhardt, H. T., Jr. 1975. Defining death: A philosophical problem for medicine and law. *American Review of Respiratory Diseases* 112:587–590.

———. 1978. Medicine and the concept of person. In T. L. Beauchamp and S. Perlin (eds.), *Ethical Issues in Death and Dying.* Englewood Cliffs, NJ: Prentice-Hall.

———. 1999. Redefining death: The mirage of consensus. In S. J. Youngner, R. M. Arnold, and R. Schapiro (eds.), *The Definition of Death: Contemporary Controversies.* Baltimore: Johns Hopkins University Press.

Erikson, E. 1956. The problem of ego identity. *Journal of the American Psychoanalytic Association* 4:56–121.

Evans, G. 1982. *The Varieties of Reference.* Oxford: Oxford University Press.

Feinberg, J. 1974. The rights of animals and unborn generations. In W. T. Blackstone (ed.), *Philosophy and Environmental Crisis.* Athens: University of Georgia Press.

Feldman, F. 1992. *Confrontations with the Reaper.* New York: Oxford University Press.

Field, D. R., Gates, E. A., Creasy, R. K., Jonsen, K. R., and Laros, R. K. 1988. Maternal brain death during pregnancy. *Journal of the American Medical Association* 260:816–822.

Fins, J. J. 2005. Rethinking disorders of consciousness: New research and its implications. *Hastings Center Report* 35(2):22–24.

Fins, J., and Plum, F. 2004. Neurological diagnosis is more than a state of mind: Diagnostic clarity and impaired consciousness (editorial). *Archives of Neurology* 61:1354–1355.

Fost, N. 1988. Organs from anencephalic infants: An idea whose time has not yet come. *Hastings Center Report* 18(5):5–10.

———. 1999. The unimportance of death. In S. J. Youngner, R. M. Arnold, and R. Schapiro (eds.), *The Definition of Death: Contemporary Controversies.* Baltimore: Johns Hopkins University Press.

Freer, J. 1984. Chronic vegetative states: Intrinsic value of biological processes. *Journal of Medicine and Philosophy* 9:395–407.

Geertz, C. 1964. The transition to humanity. In S. Tax (ed.), *Horizons of Anthropology.* Chicago: Aldine.

———. 1965. The impact of the concept of culture on the concept of man. In J. R. Platt (ed.), *New Views on the Nature of Man.* Chicago: University of Chicago Press.

———. 1966. Religion as a cultural system. In M. Banton (ed.), *Anthropological Approaches to the Study of Religion.* New York: Frederick A. Praeger.

Gergen, K. J. 1991a. *The Saturated Self: Dilemmas of Identity in Contemporary Life.* New York: Basic Books.

———. 1991b. The social construction of self-knowledge. In D. Kolak and R. Martin (eds.), *Self and Identity.* New York: Macmillan.

Gert, B. 1995. A complete definition of death. In C. Machado (ed.), *Brain Death*. Amsterdam: Elsevier.

Gervais, K. 1986. *Redefining Death*. New Haven: Yale University Press.

———. 1989. Advancing the definition of death: A philosophical essay. *Medical Humanities Review* 3(2):7–19.

Giacino, J. T., Ashwal, S., Childs, N., Cranford, R., Jennett, B., Katz, D. I., Kelly, J. P., Rosenberg, J. H., Whyte, J., Zafonte, R. D., and Zasler, N. D. 2002. The minimally conscious state: Definition and diagnostic criteria. *Neurology* 58:349–352.

Gill, C. 1990a. The human being as an ethical norm. In C. Gill (ed.), *The Person and the Human Mind*. Oxford: Oxford University Press.

Gillett, G. 1990. Consciousness, the brain and what matters. *Bioethics* 4:181–198.

———, ed. 1990b. *The Person and the Human Mind: Issues in Ancient and Modern Philosophy*. Oxford: Clarendon Press.

Gilson, E. 1940. *The Spirit of Medieval Philosophy*. New York: Charles Scribner's Sons.

———. 1956. *The Christian Philosophy of St. Thomas Aquinas*. New York: Random House.

Graham, G. 1993. *Philosophy of Mind: An Introduction*. Oxford: Blackwell.

Grant, A. C. 2000. Human brain death in perspective: Comments on the spinal dog and decapitate frog. Paper presented at the Third International Symposium on Coma and Death, February 22–25, Havana.

Green, M., and Wikler, D. 1980. Brain death and personal identity. *Philosophy and Public Affairs* 9:105–133.

Grice, H. P. [1941] 1975. Personal identity. Repr. in J. Perry (ed.), *Personal Identity*. Berkeley: University of California Press.

Guérit, J.-M. 1994. The interest of multimodality evoked potentials in the evaluation of chronic coma. *Acta Neurologica Belgica* 94:174–182.

———. 1995. Multimodality evoked potentials in the permanent vegetative state. In C. Machado (ed.), *Brain Death*. Amsterdam: Elsevier.

———. 2004. The concept of brain death. In C. Machado and D. A. Shewmon (eds.), *Brain Death and Disorders of Consciousness*. New York: Kluwer.

Guérit, J.-M., de Tourtchaninoff, M., Soveges, L., and Mahieu, P. 1993. The prognostic value of three-modality evoked potentials (TMEPs) in anoxic and traumatic coma. *Neurophysiologie Clinique* 23:209–226.

Halevy, A., and Brody, B. 1993. Brain death: Reconciling definitions, criteria, and tests. *Annals of Internal Medicine* 119:519–525.

Harré, R. 1984. *Personal Being: A Theory for Individual Psychology*. Cambridge: Harvard University Press.

———. 1989. The "self" as a theoretical concept. In M. Krausz (ed.), *Relativism: Interpretation and Confrontation*. Notre Dame, IN: University of Notre Dame Press.

Honnefelder, L. 1996. The concept of person in moral philosophy. In K. Bayertz (ed.), *Sanctity of Life and Human Dignity*. Dordrecht: Kluwer.

Howsepian, A. A. 1994. Philosophical reflections on coma. *Review of Metaphysics* 47:735–755.

———. 1996. The 1994 Multi-Society Task Force consensus statement on the persistent vegetative state: A critical analysis. *Issues in Law and Medicine* 12:3–29.

Hume, D. [1739] 1978. *A Treatise of Human Nature*, ed. L. A. Selby-Bigge, 2nd ed., rev. P. Nidditch. Oxford: Clarendon Press.

Ingvar, D. H., Brun, A., Johannson, L., and Samuelsson, S. M. 1978. Survival after severe cerebral anoxia with destruction of the cerebral cortex: The apallic syndrome. *Annals of the New York Academy of Sciences* 315:184–208; discussion, 208–214.

Jackson, F. 1982. Epiphenomenal qualia. *Philosophical Quarterly* 32:127–156.

Jennet, B., and Plum, F. 1972. Persistent vegetative state after brain damage. *Lancet* 1:734–737.

Jonas, H. 1974. Against the stream: Comments on the definition and redefinition of death. In H. Jonas, *Philosophical Essays: From Ancient Creed to Technological Man*. Englewood Cliffs, NJ: Prentice-Hall.

———. 1992. The burden and blessing of mortality. *Hastings Center Report* 22(1):34–40.

Jordan, J. 1995. Is it wrong to discriminate on the basis of homosexuality? *Journal of Social Philosophy* 26:39–52.

Joyce, R. E. 1998. Personhood and the conception event. In M. Goodman (ed.), *What Is a Person?* Clifton, NJ: Humana Press.

Joynt, R. J. 1984. A new look at death. *Journal of the American Medical Association* 252:680–682.

Kalitzkus, V. 2004. Neither dead-nor-alive: Organ donation and the paradox of "living corpses." In A. Fagan (ed.), *Making Sense of Death and Dying*. Amsterdam: Rodopi.

Kant, I. [1781/1787] 1997. *Critique of Pure Reason*, trans. P. Guyer and A. Wood. Cambridge: Cambridge University Press.

———. [1785] 1993. *Grounding for the Metaphysics of Morals*, 3rd ed., trans. J. Ellington. Indianapolis: Hackett.

Kass, L. 1971. Death as an event: A commentary on Robert Morison. *Science* 173:698–702.

Kester, C. M. 1994. Is there a person in that body? An argument for the priority of persons and the need for a new legal paradigm. *Georgetown Law Journal* 82:1643–1687.

Kirwan, C. 1970–71. How strong are the objections to essence? *Proceedings of the Aristotelian Society* 71:43–59.

Korein, J. 1997. Ontogenesis of the brain in the human organism: Definitions of life and death of the human being and person. In R. B. Edwards and E. E. Butler (eds.), *Advances in Bioethics*, vol. 2. Greenwich, CT: JAI Press.

Korsgaard, C. M. 1989. Personal identity and the unity of agency. *Philosophy and Public Affairs* 18:101–132.

Kottow, M. 1984. Ethical problems in arguments from potentiality. *Theoretical Medicine* 5:293–305.

Kripke, S. 1972. Naming and necessity. In D. Davidson and G. Harman (eds.), *Semantics of Natural Languages*. Dordrecht: Reidel.

Krpiec, M. A. 1985. *I-man: An Outline of Philosophical Anthropology*, trans. M. Lescoe. New Britain, CT: Mariel.

Kuhn, T. 1970. *The Structure of Scientific Revolutions*, 2nd ed. Chicago: University of Chicago Press.

LaFleur, W. R. 2002. From *agape* to organs: Religious difference between Japan and America in judging the ethics of the transplant. *Zygon* 37:623–642.

——. 2004. The afterlife of the corpse: How popular concerns impact upon bioethical debates in Japan. In S. Formanek and W. R. LaFleur (eds.), *Practicing the Afterlife: Perspectives from Japan*. Vienna: Verlag.

Lamb, D. 1985. *Death, Brain Death and Ethics*. New York: State University of New York.

——. 1990. *Organ Transplantation and Ethics*. London: Routledge.

——. 1992. Reversibility and death: A reply to David J. Cole. *Journal of Medical Ethics* 18: 31–33.

Langerak, E. 1979. Abortion: Listening to the middle. *Hastings Center Report* 9(1):24–28.

Laureys, S., Faymonville, M.-E., De Tiège, X , Peigneux, P., Berré, J., Moonen, G., Goldman, S., and Maquet, P. 2004. Brain function in the vegetative state. In C. Machado and D. A. Shewmon (eds.), *Brain Death and Disorders of Consciousness*. New York: Kluwer.

Leibniz. [1690] 1981. *New Essays Concerning Human Understanding*, trans. and ed. P. Remnant and J. Bennett. Cambridge: Cambridge University Press.

Lemire, R. J., Beckwith, J. B., and Warkany, J. 1978. *Anencephaly*. New York: Raven Press.

Lizza, J. P. 1991. *Metaphysical and Cultural Aspects of Persons* (Ph.D. diss., Columbia University). Ann Arbor: University Microfilms International.

——. 1993a. Multiple personality and personal identity revisited. *British Journal for the Philosophy of Science* 44:263–274.

——. 1993b. Persons and death: What's metaphysically wrong with our current statutory definition of death? *Journal of Medicine and Philosophy* 18:351–374.

——. 1999a. Death: Merely biological? (letters). *Hastings Center Report* 29(1):4.

——. 1999b. Defining death for persons and human organisms. *Theoretical Medicine and Bioethics* 20:439–453.

——. 2002. Defining death: A biological or cultural matter? In R. N. Fisher, D. T. Primozic, P. A. Day, and J. A. Thompson (eds.), *Suffering, Death, and Identity*. Amsterdam: Rodopi.

——. 2004. The conceptual basis for brain death revisited: Loss of organic integration or loss of consciousness? In C. Machado and D. A. Shewmon (eds.), *Brain Death and Disorders of Consciousness*. New York: Kluwer.

——. 2005. Potentiality, irreversibility, and death. *Journal of Medicine and Philosophy* 30:45–64.

Lock, M. 1997. The unnatural as ideology: Contesting brain death in Japan. In O. J. Asquith and A. Kalland (eds.), *Japanese Images of Nature*. Melville, NY: Curzon.

——. 1999. The problem of brain death: Japanese disputes about bodies and modernity. In S. J. Youngner, R. M. Arnold, and R. Schapiro (eds.), *The Definition of Death: Contemporary Controversies*. Baltimore: Johns Hopkins University Press.

——. 2002. *Twice Dead*. Berkeley: University of California Press.

Locke, J. [1694] 1975. *An Essay Concerning Human Understanding*, 2nd ed., ed. P. H. Nidditch. Oxford: Clarendon Press.

Lockwood, M. 1985. When does a life begin? In M. Lockwood (ed.), *Moral Dilemmas in Modern Medicine*. Oxford: Oxford University Press.

——. 1994. Identity matters. In K. W. M. Fulford, G. Gillett, and J. M. Soskice (eds.), *Med-*

icine and Moral Reasoning. Cambridge: Cambridge University Press.

Lowe, E. J. 1989. *Kinds of Being: A Study of Individuation, Identity, and the Logic of Sortal Terms.* Oxford: Basil Blackwell.

——. 1991a. Real selves: Persons as a substantial kind. In D. Cockburn (ed.), *Human Beings.* Cambridge: Cambridge University Press.

——. 1991b. Substance and selfhood. *Philosophy* 66:81–99.

Lynn, J. 1993. Are the patients who become organ donors under the Pittsburgh protocol for "non-heart-beating donors" really dead? *Kennedy Institute of Ethics Journal* 3:167–178.

Machado, C. 1995. A new definition of death based on the basic mechanism of consciousness generation in human beings. In C. Machado (ed.), *Brain Death: Proceedings of the Second International Symposium on Brain Death.* Amsterdam: Elsevier.

——. In press. The first organ transplant from a brain-dead donor. *Neurology.*

Mackie, D. 1999. Personal identity and dead people. *Philosophical Studies* 95:219–242.

Macklin, R. 1983. Personhood in the bioethics literature. *Milbank Memorial Fund Quarterly/Health and Society* 6:35–57.

Madell, G. 1981. *The Identity of the Self.* Edinburgh: Edinburgh University Press.

Malliani, D., Peterson, D. F., Bishop, V. S., and Brown, A. M. 1972. Spinal sympathetic cardiocardiac reflexes. *Circulation Research* 30:158–166.

Margolis, J. 1984. *Culture and Cultural Entities: Toward a New Unity of Science.* Dordrecht: Reidel.

Maslin, K. T. 2001. *An Introduction to the Philosophy of Mind.* Cambridge: Polity Press.

McGinn, C. 1992. *The Character of Mind.* Oxford: Oxford University Press.

McMahan, J. 1995. The metaphysics of brain death. *Bioethics* 9:91–126.

——. 2002. *The Ethics of Killing: Problems at the Margins of Life.* Oxford: Oxford University Press.

McTaggart, J. M. E. 1927. *The Nature of Existence.* Cambridge: Cambridge University Press.

Mead, G. H. 1925. The genesis of self and social control. *International Journal of Ethics* 35:251–273.

——. 1934. *Mind, Self and Society from the Standpoint of a Social Behaviorist.* Chicago: University of Chicago Press.

Medical Task Force on Anencephaly. 1990. The infant with anencephaly. *New England Journal of Medicine* 322:669–674.

Meilaender, G. 1993. *Terra es animata:* On having a life. *Hastings Center Report* 23(4):25–32.

Miles, S. 1999. Death in a technological and pluralistic culture. In S. J. Youngner, R. M. Arnold, and R. Schapiro (eds.), *The Definition of Death: Contemporary Controversies.* Baltimore: Johns Hopkins University Press.

Moore, G. E. [1903] 1993. *Principia Ethica.* Repr. Cambridge: Cambridge University Press.

Morioka, M. 2001. Reconsidering brain death: A lesson from Japan's fifteen years of experience. *Hastings Center Report* 31(4):41–46.

Morison, R. 1971. Death: Process or event? *Science* 173:694–698.

Multi-Society Task Force on PVS. 1994. Medical aspects of the persistent vegetative state: Parts 1 and 2. *New England Journal of Medicine* 330:1499–1508, 1572–1579.

Nagel, T. 1965. Physicalism. *Philosophical Review* 74:339–356.

——. 1979. What is it like to be a bat? In T. Nagel, *Mortal Questions.* Cambridge: Cambridge University Press.

———. 1986. *The View from Nowhere*. Oxford: Oxford University Press.

Noonan, J. 1968. Deciding who is human. *Natural Law Forum* 13:134–140.

Olson, E. T. 1997. *The Human Animal*. Oxford: Oxford University Press.

Orlick, R. S. 1991. Brain death, religious freedom, and public policy: New Jersey's landmark legislative initiative. *Kennedy Institute of Ethics Journal* 1:275–288.

Pallis, C. 1983. ABC of brainstem death. *British Medical Journal* 286:284–287.

Parfit, D. [1971] 1975. Personal identity. *Philosophical Review* 80(1). Repr. in J. Perry (ed.), *Personal Identity*. Berkeley: University of California Press.

———. 1986. *Reasons and Persons*. Oxford. Oxford University Press.

———. 1999. Experiences, subjects, and conceptual schemes. *Philosophical Topics* 26(1–2): 217–270.

Peabody, J. L., and Emery, J. R. 1989. Experience with anencephalic infants as prospective organ donors. *New England Journal of Medicine* 321:344–350.

Pernick, M. S. 1999. Brain death in a cultural context. In S. J. Youngner, R. M. Arnold, and R. Schapiro (eds.), *The Definition of Death: Contemporary Controversies*. Baltimore: Johns Hopkins University Press.

Persson, I. 1999. Our identity and the separability of persons and organisms. *Dialogue* 38:519–533.

———. 2002. Human death—A view from the beginning of life. *Bioethics* 16:20–32.

Plum, F. 1991. Coma and related global disturbances of the human conscious state. In A. Peters (ed.), *Cerebral Cortex*, vol. 9. New York: Plenum.

Plum, F., and Posner, F. 1980. *The Diagnosis of Stupor and Coma*, 3rd ed. Philadelphia: F. A. Davis.

Pomerance J., and Schifrin, B. S. 1987. Anencephaly and the "Baby Doe" regulations. *Pediatric Research* 21:373A.

Potts, M., Byrne, P. A., and Nilges, R., eds. 2000. *Beyond Brain Death: The Case against Brain Based Criteria for Human Death*. Dordrecht: Kluwer.

President's Commission for the Study of Ethical Problems in Medicine and Biomedical and Behavioral Research. 1981. *Defining Death: Medical, Ethical, and Legal Issues in the Determination of Death*. Washington, DC: U.S. Government Printing Office.

Prince, M. [1906] 1969. *The Dissociation of a Personality*. Repr. New York: Longmans.

Puccetti, R. 1988. Does anyone survive neocortical death? In R. M. Zaner (ed.), *Death: Beyond Whole-Brain Criteria*. Dordrecht: Kluwer.

Putnam, H. [1967] 1991. The nature of mental states. Repr. in D. M. Rosenthal (ed.), *The Nature of Mind*. New York: Oxford University Press.

———. 1970. Is semantics possible? In K. Kiefer and M. Munitz (eds.), *Languages, Beliefs and Metaphysics*. New York: State University of New York.

———. 1975. The meaning of meaning. In K. Gunderson (ed.), *Language, Mind and Knowledge* (Minnesota Studies in the Philosophy of Science, vol. 7). Minneapolis: University of Minnesota Press.

———. 1980. Brains and behavior. In N. Block (ed.), *Readings in Philosophy of Psychology*, vol. 1. Cambridge: Harvard University Press.

Quay, P. M. 1993. The hazards of brain-death statutes. *Ethics and Medics* 18(6):1–2.

Quine, W. V. O. 1960. *Word and Object*. Cambridge: MIT Press.

Ramsey, P. 1970. *The Patient as Person*. New Haven: Yale University Press.

Ray, A. C. 1985. Humanity, personhood and abortion. *International Philosophical Quarterly* 25:233–245.

Reid, T. [1895] 1969. *Essays on the Intellectual Powers of Man*. Repr. Cambridge: MIT Press.

Rolston, H. 1982. The irreversibly comatose: Respect for the subhuman in human life. *Journal of Medicine and Philosophy* 7:337–354.

Rosenberg, J. F. 1983. *Thinking Clearly about Death*. Englewood Cliffs, NJ: Prentice-Hall.

Russell, T. 2000. *Brain Death: Philosophical Concepts and Problems*. Aldershot, England: Ashgate.

Sartre, J.-P. [1942] 1994. *Being and Nothingness*, trans. H. E. Barnes. New York: Gramercy Books.

———. [1945] 1955. *No Exit*, trans. S. Gilbert. New York: Vintage Books.

———. [1946] 1970. *L'existentialisme est un humanisme*. Repr. Paris: Les Editions Nagel.

Schick, T., and Vaughn, L. 2004. *How to Think about Weird Things: Critical Thinking for a New Age*, 4th ed. Columbus, OH: McGraw-Hill.

Schiff, N., and Fins, J. 2003. Hope for "comatose" patients. *Cerebrum* 5(4):7–24.

Schöne-Seifert, B. 1999. Defining death in Germany: Brain death and its discontents. In S. J. Youngner, R. M. Arnold, and R. Schapiro (eds.), *The Definition of Death: Contemporary Controversies*. Baltimore: Johns Hopkins University Press.

Seifert, J. 1993. Is "brain death" actually death? *Monist* 76:175–202.

Shewmon, D. A. 1985. The metaphysics of brain death, persistent vegetative state, and dementia. *Thomist* 49:24–80.

———. 1987. Ethics and brain death. *New Scholasticism* 61:321–344.

———. 1988. Anencephaly: Selected medical aspects. *Hastings Center Report* 18(5):11–18.

———. 1992. Brain death: A valid theme with invalid variations, blurred by semantic ambiguity. In H. Angstwurm and I. Carrasco de Paula (eds.), *Working Group on the Determination of Brain Death and Its Relationship to Human Death*. Vatican City: Pontificia Academia Scientiarum.

———. 1997. Recovery from "brain death": A neurologist's apologia. *Linacre Quarterly* 64: 31–96.

———. 1998a. "Brainstem death," "brain death," and death: A critical reevaluation of the purported evidence. *Issues in Law and Medicine* 14:125–146.

———. 1998b. Chronic "brain death": Meta-analysis and conceptual consequences. *Neurology* 51:1538–1545.

———. 1999. Spinal shock and "brain death": Somatic pathophysiological equivalence and implications for the integrative-unity rationale. *Spinal Cord* 37:313–324.

———. 2001. The brain and somatic integration: Insights into the standard biological rationale for equating "brain death" with "death." *Journal of Medicine and Philosophy* 26:457–478.

———. 2004a. The ABC of PVS. In C. Machado and D. A. Shewmon (eds.), *Brain Death and Disorders of Consciousness*. New York: Kluwer.

———. 2004b. The "critical organ" for the "organism as a whole": Lessons from the lowly spinal cord. In C. Machado and D. A. Shewmon (eds.), *Brain Death and Disorders of Con-*

sciousness. New York: Kluwer.

Shewmon, D. A., Holmes, G. L., and Byrne, P. A. 1999. Consciousness in congenitally decorticate children: "Developmental vegetative state" as self-fulfilling prophecy. *Developmental Medicine and Child Neurology* 41:364–374.

Shewmon, D. A., and Shewmon, E. S. 2004. The semiotics of death and its medical implications. In C. Machado and D. A. Shewmon (eds.), *Brain Death and Disorders of Consciousness.* New York: Kluwer.

Shinnar, S., and Arras, J. 1989. Ethical issues in the use of anencephalic infants as organ donors. *Neurologic Clinics* 7:729–743.

Shoemaker, S. 1968. Self-reference and self-awareness. *Journal of Philosophy* 65:555–567.

———. 1970. Persons and their pasts. *American Philosophical Quarterly* 7:269–285.

Shoemaker, S., and Swinburne, R. 1984. *Personal Identity.* Oxford: Basil Blackwell.

Smith, J. 1982. Letter to the editor. *Hastings Center Report* 12(6):45–46.

Smith, R. E., ed. 1989. *Critical Issues in Contemporary Health Care: Proceedings of the Eighth Bishops' Workshop, Dallas, Texas.* Braintree, MA: Pope John Center.

Snowdon, P. F. 1990. Person, animals and ourselves. In C. Gill (ed.), *The Person and the Human Mind: Issues in Ancient and Modern Philosophy.* Oxford: Clarendon Press.

———. 1991. Personal identity and brain transplants. In D. Cockburn (ed.), *Human Beings.* Cambridge: Cambridge University Press.

Strawson, G. 1994. *Mental Reality.* Cambridge: MIT Press.

Strawson, P. F. [1958] 1991. Persons. In H. Feigl, M. Scriven, and G. Maxwell (eds.), *Concepts, Theories, and the Mind-Body Problem* (Minnesota Studies in the Philosophy of Science, vol. 2). Minneapolis: University of Minnesota Press. Repr. in D. M. Rosenthal (ed.), *The Nature of Mind.* New York: Oxford University Press.

———. 1959. *Individuals.* London: Methuen.

Task Force on Death and Dying of the Institute of Society, Ethics, and the Life Sciences. 1972. Refinements in criteria for the determination of death: An appraisal. *Journal of the American Medical Association* 221:48–53.

Taylor, R. M. 1997. Re-examining the definition and criteria of death. *Seminars in Neurology* 17:265–270.

Thomson, J. J. 1987. People and their bodies. In J. Dancy (ed.), *Reading Parfit.* Malden, MA: Blackwell.

Tomlinson, T. 1984. The conservative use of the brain-death criterion—a critique. *Journal of Medicine and Philosophy* 9:377–393.

———. 1993. The irreversibility of death: Reply to Cole. *Kennedy Institute of Ethics Journal* 3:157–165.

Truog, R. D. 1997. Is it time to abandon brain death? *Hastings Center Report* 27(1):29–37.

Truog, R. D., and Fackler, J. C. 1992. Rethinking brain death. *Critical Care Medicine* 20:1705–1713.

Unger, P. 1990. *Identity, Consciousness and Value.* New York: Oxford University Press.

Veatch, R. M. 1972. Brain death: Welcome definition . . . or dangerous judgment? *Hastings Center Report* 2(5):11–13.

———. 1975. The whole-brain oriented concept of death: An outmoded philosophical formulation. *Journal of Thanatology* 3:13–30.

——. 1976. *Death, Dying and the Biological Revolution: Our Last Quest for Responsibility.* New Haven: Yale University Press.

——. 1978. Defining death anew: Technical and ethical problems. In T. L. Beauchamp and S. Perlin (eds.), *Ethical Issues in Death and Dying.* Englewood Cliffs, NJ: Prentice-Hall.

——. 1982. Maternal brain death: An ethicist's thoughts. *Journal of the American Medical Association* 248:1102–1103.

——. 1988. Whole-brain, neocortical, and higher brain related concepts. In R. M. Zaner (ed.), *Death: Beyond Whole-Brain Criteria.* Dordrecht: Kluwer.

——. 1992. Brain death and slippery slopes. *Journal of Clinical Ethics* 3:181–187.

——. 1993. The impending collapse of the whole-brain definition of death. *Hastings Center Report* 23(4):18–24.

——. 1999. The conscience clause: How much individual choice in defining death can our society tolerate? In S. J. Youngner, R. M. Arnold, and R. Schapiro (eds.), *The Definition of Death: Contemporary Controversies.* Baltimore: Johns Hopkins University Press.

Wallace, W. A. 1995. St. Thomas on the beginning and ending of human life. In A. Vari (ed.), *Sanctus Thomas de Aquino Doctor Hodiernae Humanitatis* (Studi Tomistici 58) Vatican City: Libreria Editrice Vaticana. Available at www.nd.edu/Departments/Maritain/ti/wallace3.htm.

Walton, D. 1980. *Brain Death: Ethical Considerations.* West Lafayette, IN: Purdue University Press.

Warren, M. 2000. *Moral Status: Obligations to Persons and Other Living Things.* Oxford: Oxford University Press.

Wartofsky, M. 1988. Beyond a whole-brain definition of death: Reconsidering the metaphysics of death. In R. M. Zaner (ed.), *Death: Beyond Whole-Brain Criteria.* Dordrecht: Kluwer.

White, R. J., Wolin, L. R., Masopust, L., Taslitz, N., and Verdura, J. 1971. Cephalic exchange transplantation in the monkey. *Surgery* 70:135–139.

White, S. 1989. Metapsychological relativism and the self. *Journal of Philosophy* 86:298–323.

Wiggins, D. 1974. Essentialism, continuity, and identity. *Synthese* 28:321–359.

——. 1976. The *de re* "must": A note on the logical form of essentialist claims. In G. Evans and J. McDowell (eds.), *Truth and Meaning: Essays in Semantics.* Oxford: Oxford University Press.

——. 1980. *Sameness and Substance.* Cambridge: Harvard University Press.

——. 1987. The person as object of science, as subject of experience, and as the locus of value. In A. Peacocke and G. Gillet (eds.), *Persons and Personality: A Contemporary Inquiry.* Oxford: Oxford University Press.

——. 2001. *Sameness and Substance Renewed.* Cambridge: Cambridge University Press.

Wikler, D. 1995. Who defines death? Medical, legal and philosophical perspectives. In C. Machado (ed.), *Brain Death: Proceedings of the Second International Symposium on Brain Death.* Amsterdam: Elsevier.

Wilkes, K. 1981. Multiple personality and personal identity. *British Journal for the Philosophy of Science* 32:331–348.

Williams, B. [1970] 1973. The self and the future. *Philosophical Review* 59. Repr. in B. Williams,

Problems of the Self. Cambridge: Cambridge University Press.

Wittgenstein, L. 1953. *Philosophical Investigations,* trans. G. E. M. Anscombe. Oxford: Blackwell.

Youngner, S. J., Arnold, R. M., and Schapiro R., eds., 1999. *The Definition of Death: Contemporary Controversies.* Baltimore: Johns Hopkins University Press.

Younger, S., and Bartlett. E. 1983. Human death and high technology: The failure of the whole-brain formulations. *Annals of Internal Medicine* 99:252–258.

Zaner, R. M., ed. 1988. *Death: Beyond Whole-Brain Criteria* (Philosophy and Medicine, vol. 31, ed. T. J. Engelhardt and S. F. Spicker). Dordrecht: Kluwer.

Index